Keratitis - Current Perspectives

Edited by Anna Nowińska

Published in London, United Kingdom

Keratitis - Current Perspectives
http://dx.doi.org/10.5772/intechopen.107689
Edited by Anna Nowińska

Contributors
Alberto Haber Olguin, Guillermo Raúl Vera Duarte, Luis Antonio García Padilla, Patricia R do Prado, Fernanda R. E Gimenes, Marta Świerczyńska, Agnieszka Tronina, Ewa Mrukwa-Kominek, Lional Raj Daniel Raj Ponniah, Edyta Chlasta-Twardzik, Anna Nowińska, Cansu Yuksel Elgin

First published in London, United Kingdom, 2024 by IntechOpen
IntechOpen is the global imprint of INTECHOPEN LIMITED, registered in England and Wales, registration number: 11086078, 5 Princes Gate Court, London, SW7 2QJ, United Kingdom

British Library Cataloguing-in-Publication Data
A catalogue record for this book is available from the British Library

Additional hard and PDF copies can be obtained from orders@intechopen.com

Keratitis - Current Perspectives
Edited by Anna Nowińska
p. cm.
Print ISBN 978-1-83768-340-6
Online ISBN 978-1-83768-341-3
eBook (PDF) ISBN 978-1-83768-772-5

For EU product safety concerns:
IN TECH d.o.o., Prolaz Marije Krucifikse Kozulić 3, 51000 Rijeka, Croatia,
info@intechopen.com or visit our website at intechopen.com.

Meet the editor

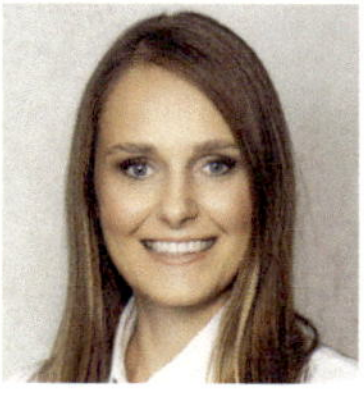

Prof. Anna Nowinska is an ophthalmic microsurgeon and a clinician-scientist, who performs cataract and vitreoretinal surgeries and conducts basic science research on ocular surface diseases as well as retinal diseases and multimodal retinal and corneal imaging. She is an associate professor at the Medical University of Silesia, Poland. She was granted the Polish Health Minister Scholarship for achievements in science. In 2015–2019, Dr. Nowinska was the principal investigator of the National Science Center grant, "Phenotype-genotype analysis of patients with corneal dystrophies originating from Polish population." Her work has led to numerous peer-reviewed publications, review articles, and presentations nationally and internationally.

Contents

Preface **IX**

Section 1
Infectious Keratitis **1**

Chapter 1 **3**
Bacterial Keratitis
by Edyta Chlasta-Twardzik and Anna Nowińska

Chapter 2 **23**
Infectious Keratitis after Surgery
by Alberto Haber Olguin, Guillermo Raúl Vera Duarte and Luis Antonio García Padilla

Chapter 3 **35**
Alternative Treatment Approaches in Bacterial Keratitis
by Lional Raj Daniel Raj Ponniah

Section 2
Non-Infectious Keratitis **47**

Chapter 4 **49**
Peripheral Ulcerative Keratitis Associated with Autoimmune Diseases
by Marta Świerczyńska, Agnieszka Tronina and Ewa Mrukwa-Kominek

Chapter 5 **77**
Dry Eye Disease: Chronic Ocular Surface Inflammation
by Anna Nowińska

Section 3
Miscellaneous **91**

Chapter 6 **93**
Challenges of the Intraocular Pressure Measurements in the Keratitis
by Cansu Yuksel Elgin

Chapter 7 105
Prevention of Corneal Injury in Critically Ill Sedated and Mechanically Ventilated Patients: Theoretical and Evidence-Based Practice
by Patricia R. do Prado and Fernanda R.E. Gimenes

Preface

This book provides a comprehensive overview of current ocular diagnostic methods, including their theoretical basis, practical approach, and usage in clinical practice, as well as recent advances in keratitis treatment methods.

The authors of the 2019 World Health Organization Report on Vision reported that at least 2.2 billion people globally have vision impairment; of these, at least one billion have an issue that could have been treated or prevented. Keratitis is still one of the leading causes of blindness in the world. In most cases, corneal diseases represent preventable or treatable ophthalmic diseases, therefore a comprehensive knowledge of epidemiology, causes, accurate diagnosis, and treatment of the multiple forms of keratitis is crucial in clinical practice.

The book underlines the role of ocular surface system homeostasis. The ocular surface system is composed of the surface and glandular epithelia of the cornea, conjunctiva, lacrimal gland, accessory lacrimal glands, and meibomian gland, and their apical (tears) and basal (connective tissue) matrices, the eyelashes with their associated glands of Moll and Zeis, those components of the eyelids responsible for the blink, and the nasolacrimal duct. All components of this vital system are linked functionally by continuity of the epithelia, by innervation, and by the endocrine, vascular, and immune systems. Ocular surface system homeostasis encompasses the causes, clinical forms, and methods of treatment of multiple diseases including non-infectious and infectious keratitis. Keratitis is a disease of many etiological factors, multiple forms, and different severity; therefore management and therapeutic options should be implemented according to disease form and severity.

The book's first section, discusses the practical approach to treating keratitis. Chapter 1 "Bacterial Keratitis" discusses bacterial keratitis. Chapter 2 "Infectious Keratitis after Surgery" examines potential infectious complications after refractive surgeries. Chapter 3 "Alternative Treatment Approaches in Bacterial Keratitis" reviews novel drug delivery systems, such as contact lenses for constant drug delivery, microemulsions, plasma and phage therapy, cross-linking, thymosin beta 4, novel implantable sustained-release antibacterial disc, and intrastromal injections with antibiotic agents.

The second section covers non-infectious keratitis. Chapter 4 "Peripheral Ulcerative Keratitis Associated with Autoimmune Diseases" presents a stepwise approach to diagnosing and treating peripheral ulcerative keratitis. Chapter 5 "Dry Eye Disease: Chronic Ocular Surface Inflammation" examines the role of ocular surface inflammation in dry eye disease pathogenesis.

The last book section discusses two essential issues related to keratitis: intraocular pressure measurements in Chapter 6 "Challenges of the Intraocular Pressure Measurements in the Keratitis" and prevention of corneal injury in sedated and mechanically ventilated patients in Chapter 7 "Prevention of Corneal Injury in Critically Ill Sedated and Mechanically Ventilated Patients: Theoretical and Evidence-Based Practice".

Anna Nowińska
Chair and Department of Ophthalmology,
Faculty of Medical Sciences in Zabrze,
Medical University of Silesia,
Katowice, Poland

Section 1

Infectious Keratitis

Chapter 1

Bacterial Keratitis

Edyta Chlasta-Twardzik and Anna Nowińska

Abstract

Bacterial keratitis is a disease prevalent in the underdeveloped and developing worlds and is a significant cause of vision-threatening keratitis across the globe. Early and exact diagnosis, accurate treatment, and regular follow-up are key determinants of success in these cases and allow to prevent serious complications and ensure optimal patient outcomes. This chapter provides a comprehensive overview of the causes, symptoms, diagnosis, and management of bacterial keratitis. The importance of accurate diagnosis based on culture of corneal scraping, and smear examinations, as well as with the use of diagnostic tools, such as confocal microscopy is highlighted. Treatment options, including medical treatment and surgical interventions, are discussed in detail. Moreover, the chapter provides insights into the latest research and developments including new treatments. It also highlights the need for ongoing monitoring, regular follow-up, and good compliance between patient and doctor to ensure optimal patient outcomes. The patient must be educated to avoid risk factors. The superficial ulcer usually responds well to medical management, whereas deeper non-resolving ulcers require therapeutic penetrating keratoplasty for globe salvage. Overall, this chapter serves as an important resource for clinicians, researchers, and healthcare professionals, providing valuable information on the diagnosis and management of bacterial keratitis.

Keywords: bacterial keratitis, bacterial corneal ulcer, corneal infection, infectious keratitis, medical therapy

1. Introduction

Infectious keratitis (IK) is a condition that can occur as a consequence of pathogen invasion into the tissue or as an autoimmune disease accompanying systemic diseases. IK is a corneal infection also known as corneal opacity or corneal ulcer. IK represents the fifth leading cause of blindness globally, accounting for ~3.2% of all cases [1]. It is estimated to be responsible for 1.5–2.0 million cases of unilateral blindness annually [2]. According to WHO, 1.9 million people have corneal blindness due to the opacification of the cornea, which accounts for about 5% of the total patients who have blindness [3]. Corneal Opacity accounts for 3.46% of global blindness and 1.65% of global blindness and visual impairment. Infectious keratitis can be divided into microbial keratitis, including bacteria, fungi, or parasites and viral keratitis, including herpes viruses [4]. Microbial keratitis is an infectious disease of the eye, in which the cornea is inflamed. Bacteria are most concerning due to rapidly progressive vision-threatening keratitis with irreversible visual sequelae. The localization of corneal inflammation is important, and acute inflammations usually affect the central part of the tissue, while peripherally located forms of corneal inflammation are more often of prolonged inflammation with an etiology that is difficult to clearly determine.

Bacterial keratitis (BK) is the most common type among all types of infectious keratitis. BK accounts for approximately 65–90% of all microbial keratitis [5]. BK rarely occurs in the healthy eye because of the human cornea's natural anatomical barrier to infection. BK is caused by varied bacterial species, and it can be an acute, chronic, or transient infectious process of the cornea. BK is one of the most common causes of visual impairment in working-age adults. BK is one of the most serious ocular infections, and it can progress rapidly and may lead to serious complications including vision-threatening keratitis. Acute keratitis may progress with tissue necrosis and its perforation within even several dozen hours. When analyzing the causes of bacterial keratitis, a number of external factors should be taken into consideration such as climate, geographical zone, level of hygiene, patient's workplace, use of contact lenses, and the endemic occurrence of various eye diseases. Whereas local factors include medical history, especially dry eye syndrome, other local disorders of the eye surface, especially those affecting the epithelium and the human margin, surgical procedures, or the presence of sutures. The diagnosis of BK is based on clinical and microbiological evaluation. Thus, to avoid a serious complication early and immediate medical treatment is needed. Recently, in the past few decades have seen increasing contact lens users, resulting in proportionately increased of bacterial keratitis and corneal ulcers [6].

2. Etiology

The surface of the human eye has not only excellent and efficient defense mechanisms protecting against the invasion of pathogens but also against bacteria existing on the surface of the conjunctiva and skin. The main barriers protect to microbial infection are anatomical barriers (eyelids, intact conjunctiva, corneal epithelium, and tear film) and antimicrobial barriers (tear film constituents IgA, complement components, lactoferrin, lysozymes, and conjunctiva-associated lymphoid tissue (CALT)) [7]. These barriers could be disrupted and predispose to infection. Every break in the continuity of the epithelium may predispose to pathogen invasion into the cornea. Every minor injury, foreign body, or wound can be a trigger factor of inflammation.

The bacterial spectrum from different areas or periods is widely reported in the literature, and those differences could be associated with weather, rural vs. urban area, and etiology of keratitis. The most common pathogens that are associated with bacterial keratitis include *Staphylococcus aureus*, Coagulase-negative staphylococci, *Staphylococcus epidermidis*, *Streptococcus pneumoniae*, *Pseudomonas aeruginosa*, and species of the *Enterobacteriaceae* family [8]. This group of bacteria is characterized a good adherence to the epithelium and to the surface of contact lenses. *Staphylococcus epidermidis* and *Staphylococcus fusarium* species are the most commonly implicated in polymicrobial keratitis with trauma being the most common inciting factor [9]. The bacterial species that can penetrate the intact corneal epithelium are *Neisseria gonorrhoeae*, *Corynebacterium diphtheriae*, *Hemophilus aegyptius*, and *Listeria monocytogenes* [10].

Contact lens use is one of the major causes of bacterial keratitis in developed countries, whereas trauma is the main risk factor in developing countries [11, 12]. The etiology of CL-related keratitis is most commonly associated with *Pseudomonas aeruginosa* and *Acanthamoeba* species. These two types of bacteria are free-living microorganisms that are omnipresent in the environment, including water and CL solutions [13]. The risk factors of CL-related IK include: tear recession under

CL, reduction of tear exchange during blinking, and reduced corneal epithelial cell desquamation. These result in accumulation and adherence of microbes to the cornea and provide to increase risk of IK. Other local predisposing risk factors for BK are ocular surface disease (OSD), including dry eyes, corneal suture-related infection, abnormalities of eyelid anatomy and function, trichiasis, blepharitis, chronic dacryocystitis, ectropion, entropion conjunctivitis, lagophthalmos neurotrophic keratopathy, recurrent corneal erosions, epithelial defect, secondary bacterial keratitis after viral keratitis, bullous keratopathy, corneal disease, previous keratitis, xerophthalmia, blepharoconjunctivitis, fifth and seventh cranial nerve palsy. Other risk factors include mechanical or thermal injury, ocular trauma, foreign body injury, previous ocular or eyelid surgery, immunosuppression, previous corticosteroids and NSAIDs [14, 15]. Risk factors predisposing to BK are the systemic conditions such as diabetes mellitus, atopic dermatitis, connective tissue or autoimmune pathologies, Steven-Johnson syndrome (SJS), ocular mucous membrane pemphigoid (OMMP), compromised immune systems, graft-versus-host disease, immunosuppression (AIDS), chronic alcoholism, and malnourishment [16].

3. Epidemiology

The most common causative factor of IK in most regions is bacteria. BK represents the following percentage of IK, including the UK (91–93%) [17, 18], Middle East (91.8%) [19], North America (86–92%) [20], South America (79–88%) [21], and Australasia (93–100%) [22]. In the USA, the incidence of MK is 71tousends cases per year USA [23]. There is a huge disproportion in the incidence of BK between developing and developed countries. This disparity of prevalence and incidence of BK is because of differences in geographical location and environmental and climate risk factors. The contact lens' users are also significant. The pathogenesis of CL-related corneal inflammation is complex and multifactorial. CL-related IK occurs particularly in the developed and industrialized countries have been a higher frequency of contact lens' users, and as a result, there is a higher rate of contact lens-related bacterial keratitis [24, 25]. It is commonly believed that CL-related IK is caused by superficial injury secondary to CL wear. However, there are several studies in which have been shown that the presence or absence of epithelial injury did not influence the risk or severity of IK [26]. As we mentioned before, *Pseudomonas keratitis* is one of the most common causes of BK, especially in the developed countries where there is increased prevalence of CL wear.

4. Pathophysiology

The process of bacterial keratitis initiates once the epithelial is breached by any *means*. When a critical number of pathogens is exceeded, defense mechanisms fail and the stroma of the cornea is invaded by bacteria. This is facilitated by breaking the continuity of the epithelium. Only a small number of bacteria are able to break the continuous epithelium, these are gonorrhea, *Corynebacterium diphtheria*, *Corynebacterium aegyptian*, *Listeria*, and *Shigella*.

The development of bacterial keratitis progresses through four stages: stage of progressive infiltration, stage of active ulceration, stage of regression, and stage of cicatrization [27].

An important feature that determines pathogenicity is the ability of the bacterium to produce enzymes that facilitate penetration into tissues and their destruction. *Pseudomonas aeruginosa*, which produces protease, trypsin, elastase, and hemolysin, is particularly dangerous. These enzymes lead to rapidly progressing liquefied necrosis of the tissue. This bacterium should always be considered and differential as a cause of acute keratitis in CL users [25, 26, 28]. Another mechanism of tissue damage by the bacteria is the production of toxins in the form of exotoxins and the release of endotoxins after cell death that damage host cells [28]. The final course of bacterial keratitis is dependent on the virulence of the offending bacteria, host defensive mechanisms, and the treatment received.

5. Clinical features

The development of a bacterial corneal inflammation may occur as a number of clinical features. We should keep in mind that in BK signs are more common than symptoms. The common symptoms of bacterial ulcers include worsening of vision, pain, foreign body sensation, redness, watering, mucopurulent or purulent discharge, and photophobia. The various signs include lid edema, blepharospasm, mucopurulent or purulent discharge, conjunctival hyperemia and chemosis, circumcorneal congestion, epithelial defect, stromal edema and infiltrate, full-thickness infiltrate, Descemet membrane folds, hypopyon, exudates in the anterior chamber, anterior uveitis, posterior synechiae, muddy iris, and small ischemic pupil [28].

In most cases of BK, there is an epithelial defect with hyperemia and exudate mucopurulent discharge accompanied by sudden severe eye pain and photophobia. Corneal infiltrate, which causes loss of tissue transparency, as a result leads to decreased visual acuity. Inflammatory exudate may also occur in the anterior chamber of the eye and penetrate deep into the eye tissues, including the posterior segment of the eye. Such an acute course of infection with the involvement of the posterior segment of the eye occurs mainly in people with impaired immune response, using long-term steroid therapy, after eye surgery or trauma, especially after trauma with organic material. The course of the disease, as well as ocular signs and symptoms depends on the virulence of the pathogen. The increased severity of the corneal ulcer the poorer treatment results. Depending on the severity of signs and symptoms, as well as the rate of progression, BK inflammation can be divided into mild, moderate, and severe. Mild corneal ulcers <2 mm in size with the depth of the ulcer $<20\%$ or 100 μm corneal thickness that may be accompanied by superficial infiltrates near the ulcer. Moderate corneal ulcers range between 2 and 5 mm in size, depth of 20–50% (100–275 μm) of the cornea, accompanied by dense infiltrates, including the mid stroma. Severe ulcers ≥ 5 mm, with a depth of more than 50% (>275 μm), accompanied by dense infiltrates, include the deep layers of the corneal stroma [11, 22, 29].

The clinical features of corneal infiltration also depend on the type of pathogen that caused BK. Bacterial corneal ulceration can occure very often in the form of a single corneal infiltrate with a sharp epithelial demarcation, with a dense, purulent infiltration of the corneal stroma with indistinct borders accompanied by corneal edema. The main factors, which favor the development of bacterial ulcers with hypopyon, include the host tissue's resistance, as well as the bacteria's virulence. They occur generally in old, debilitated, malnourished, and with immunodeficiency patients.

BK caused by gram-positive bacteria, especially cocci, is characterized by a benign course with limited tissue infiltration located superficially with slight corneal swelling. They occur in patients with dry eye syndrome, blepharitis, and rosacea. They are characterized by slow progression, but if left untreated, they can even lead to corneal perforation. Sufficient prophylaxis is the treatment of ocular surface disorders [28]. Gram-negative bacteria produce enzymes that quickly damage tissue. They are characterized by rapid progression and the lack or delayed implementation of treatment leads to complete destruction of the cornea, sclera, iris, and even loss of the eyeball. *Pseudomonas aeruginosa* usually progresses rapidly with stromal melt and necrosis, ring infiltrate, hypopyon, anterior chamber cells and flare, endothelial plaque, and later descemetocele formation or perforation [28, 30]. *Pseudomonas aeruginosa* is more common in CL-wear patients as this bacterium becomes more pathogenic in biofilm associated with the contact lens [13, 25, 26, 30]. Some bacteria cause characteristic changes in the corneal stroma, which is helpful in making the diagnosis. Streptococci cause limited infiltrates, the descent of which is crystalline keratopathy. Gram-negative bacteria, such as *Klebsiella*, *Proteus*, *Listeria*, *Streptococcus*, and *Pseudomonas*, favor the appearance of the characteristic annular shape infiltrates of the cornea [28].

6. Diagnostic tests

In the case of a diagnostic process of BK, an interview with the patient and microbiological tests are important. The clinical appearance of the infection is not a reliable factor indicating the causative pathogen. Routine proceeding should be the collection of material for culture and preparation of direct material. In patients wearing contact lenses, the contact lens itself may provide key information about the pathogen. The corneal ulcer should be cultured for the identification of the causal organism and make an antibiogram for achieve an antibiotic susceptibility before commencing antimicrobial therapy [31]. Based on the American Academy of Ophthalmology, it is still recommended to perform the first culture and/or smears in the following situations [9]:

- Infiltrates located in the central part of the cornea or large corneal infiltrate and/or associated with significant stromal involvement or melting
- Infiltrates involved a large area of the cornea (> 2 mm)
- Significant multiple infiltrates in different area of the cornea
- Previous history of corneal surgeries
- Chronic or unresponsive keratitis to broad-spectrum antibiotics therapy
- Atypical clinical features suggesting fungal, amoebic, or mycobacterial keratitis

6.1 Microbiology evaluation

The microbiological evaluation consists of smear examination and culture of corneal scrapings into several media to grow organisms for identification [32]. Culture is the only way to determine, which antibiotics the pathogenetic agent is susceptible to. In the case of sight-threatening keratitis, the culture is an indispensable diagnostic tool. The results of culture allow to shorten the duration of treatment and avoid unnecessary drug use. The efficiency of corneal cultures and smears is much higher if done before antibiotic treatment is initiated. However, when a patient previously used antibiotics, antibiotic therapy should be discontinued and scraping can be delayed for 12–24 hours to improve test performance. Lately, calcium alginate swabs with trypticase soy broth have been employed to obtain corneal specimens for obtaining a higher yield of bacteria [33]. When obtaining specimens, we should be very careful in the case of descemetocele, deep stromal keratitis, or corneal melting. The corneal ulcer samples are performed under topical anesthesia (i.e., 1% lignocaine, 0.5% proparacaine, or proxymetacaine 0.5%). There should be preferred preservative-free formulation because preservative may lower the bacterial viability for culture. Before performing scraping, dead and necrotic tissue and loose mucus are removed from the ulcer surface. Then, the corneal ulcer samples are collected from the area of corneal infiltration (the margin and the base of the ulcer) using a disposable number 11 or 15 Bard-Parker blade or typically 25-gauge or 26 G bent hypodermic needle or sterile kimura or platinum spatula. The first samples are placed on glass slides for staining, and then onto the media for culture [12, 33, 34]. The obtained material is smeared onto one or two glass slides for microscopic evaluation along with a gram stain. Gram staining detects the type of organism in 60–75% of bacterial cases, and it is beneficial providing results in 5 minutes [12, 31]. Repeat scraping is performed, and the sample is placed on various culture media that should be taken from the fridge and left for 1 h to reach room temperature. Various stains used for bacteria and various culture media for bacteria are shown in **Tables 1** and **2** [35].

According to literature data from around the world, the positive culture rate from corneal scrapes ranges from 38 to 66% [36–42]. When smear and culture results are negative two times, and there is a clinical progression of ulcer despite the best antibacterial therapy a corneal biopsy can be performed. It is obtained with the help of a dermal trephine or freehand dissection, and the specimen is divided into two halves to

Gram stain	Gram-positive bacteria appear purple and gram-negative as pink
Acridine orange	Bacteria appear as yellow-green
Acid Fast	Mycobacterium appear as pink

Table 1.
Various stains used for bacteria.

Blood agar (35 degrees)	*Aerobic* and facultative *anaerobic* bacteria
Chocolate agar (35 degrees)	*Aerobic*, *anaerobic*, *Neisseria*, *Moraxella* and *Haemophilus*
Thioglycolate broth (35 degrees)	*Aerobic* bacteria and *Anaerobic* bacteria
Sabouraud's dextrose agar (Room temperature)	*Nocardia*
Brain heart infusion broth (Room temperature)	*Nocardia*
Middlebrook Cohn agar (35 degree with 3 to 10% CO_2)	*Mycobacterium* and *Nocardia*
Cooked meat broth (35 degrees)	*Anaerobic* bacteria
Thayer martin blood agar (35 degrees)	*Neisseria*
Lowenstein Jensen media (35 degrees with 3 to 10% CO_2)	*Mycobacterium* species

Table 2.
Various culture media for bacteria.

allow histopathological and microbiological analysis [9, 43]. Conjunctival swab culture (calcium alginate swabs give the best results) may be another important additional diagnostic method in severe cases when culture growth is negative [44]. Anterior chamber paracentesis is another needed diagnostic method, which is performed in the case of negative scraping culture, or there is a progression of ulcer despite the best antibacterial therapy. A 0.1 to 0.2 ml sample is obtained with the help of a 25 G needle by a side port [45]. In addition to corneal scrapping, it is worth to obtain culture from contact lenses, liquids, and containers for lenses and from other potential sources of infection, for example, from inflamed eyelids. A relationship has been demonstrated between cultures of the abovementioned sources and corneal scraping [46]. We should keep in mind, that as interpreting results caution is needed because most eyelid and ocular surface commensal organisms are gram-positive and likely to contaminate the sample [47].

6.2 Polymerase chain reaction test

The polymerase chain reaction (PCR) test is another test used in the diagnosis of microbial keratitis. This is a molecular technique for the detection and analysis of specific DNA sequences, consisting of repeated cycles of denaturation, amplification, and replication, in which segments of DNA are continuously multiplied to enable their detection [48]. The advantages of PCR, including sensitivity, speed, and cost-effectiveness relative to culture and staining. It also gives an ability to quickly differentiate bacterial and fungal ulcers. It also gives a possibility to detect of slow-growing bacteria and organisms that are difficult to cultivate or identify with traditional microbiological methods [49–51]. This technology also has an important role in diagnosing rare organisms, such as atypical mycobacteria and Nocardia species [52]. There are also some disadvantages, including the high rate of false positive errors from commensal contaminants or dead bacteria, lower specificity compared with culture and staining, difficulty to interpret results and treating by clinician, more expensive procedure, and less cost-effective when performed with a multi-organisms PCR approach, and is not readily available at all sites [49–51].

6.3 *In vivo* confocal microscopy (IVCM)

In vivo confocal microscopy (IVMC) is a noninvasive examination that shows real-time visualization of corneal layers and structures and pathological agents within the corneal tissue. The advantages of IVCM are repeatability, rapidity, and noninvasiveness, thus also being useful in monitoring the therapy. The high sensitivity and specificity of IVCM is a valuable adjuvant to the other diagnostic assays. Thanks to immediate results obtained after conducted rapid in vivo corneal examination, it allows the prompt beginning of appropriate treatment, and some authors recommend its use as a very good diagnostic tool early in the course of the disease [53]. IVCM is also useful appreciate the depth of the infection in the corneal stroma, what is an important prognostic factor of IK [54]. However, there are some disadvantages that include patient collaboration and patience are required during testing, the high price of the device, lack of availability at all sites, and difficulty in both acquiring and interpreting images by non-experienced clinician [54]. When we have access to IVCM, we should always consider to perform this examination in the following clinical situations: deeply situated infiltrates, where corneal scrapes do not have access to avoid invasive corneal biopsy, MK occurring after corneal surgery (i.e., intracorneal implants, refractive surgery), lack of the positive results in current treatment with antifungal or anti-*Acanthamoeba* spp. therapy, when actively proliferating microorganisms are found in the profound, inaccessible corneal stroma [53, 54]. IVCM is highly sensitive and specific, and thus is very useful in cases of fungal or *Acanthamoeba keratitis*. As for nowadays, IVCM should be used alongside cultures and smears. Other new diagnostic modalities, such as immunohistochemistry, enzyme immunoassay, and radioimmunoassay, are recent upcoming modalities but still have a limited role in diagnosing BK [55].

7. Treatment

The most important goal of medical treatment is to preserve vision and maintain corneal transparency. The medical treatment of a BK should be started promptly before the etiological agent is known. The initial treatment is usually empiric as culture results can take over 48 hours, and the infection can progress rapidly without treatment. All patients should start on broad-spectrum antibiotic therapy, covering both gram-positive and negative bacteria after obtaining the smear results. Due to the high probability of bacterial etiology, in doubtful cases of fungal and viral infections, an antibiotic is also used in addition to drugs against these pathogens. In the case of severe infections characterized by heterogeneous bacterial flora or in the case of larger and deep stromal ulcers, it usually prompts the use of two broad-spectrum antibiotics to prevent irreversible vision-threatening sequelae. The antibiogram, which we obtain a few days after the implementation of empirical treatment, allows to verify the initial diagnosis and decide whether to continue or modify the initial treatment. Treatment should be changed based on the results of culture and susceptibility testing. Different indications in the antibiogram should not lead to a change in the treatment profile if there is observed a clinical improvement after the implementation of empirical treatment [12].

7.1 Antibiotics

The main goal of treatment is broad-spectrum topical antibiotics, which should be used until culture results are available. The basis of the therapy is obtaining high concentrations of antibiotics within the infected tissue. For severe BK, an initial frequent dosage every 5–15 min is recommended. Thus, the eye drops are applied even hourly in the first day of therapy. At the beginning of therapy, in order to increase the effectiveness of the therapy, eye drops with a higher concentration of the drug (fortified eye drops) are often used than in commercial usage.

The main group of antibiotics used in bacterial keratitis is fluoroquinolones. Fluoroquinolones are the group of antibiotics that provide excellent tissue penetration, quickly reaching high concentrations within tissues and have a broad spectrum of bactericidal activity. There are four generations of fluoroquinolones, of which the broadest spectrum of activity has the fourth generation of fluoroquinolones, including moxifloxacin and gatifloxacin. Within the third generation, the commercially available drug is levofloxacin. Treatment can also be carried out using second-generation drugs, that is, which is the drug of choice in gonorrhea infections. The AAO BK Preferred Practice Pattern, the Royal College of Ophthalmologists Focus, UK initially recommends monotherapy with fluoroquinolones (ciprofloxacin 3 mg/ml, ofloxacin 3 mg/ml, moxifloxacin 5 mg/ml, levofloxacin 15 mg/ml, gatifloxacin 3 mg/ml, or besifloxacin 6 mg/ml). An alternative includes a combination of cephalosporin or vancomycin plus and an aminoglycoside. Vancomycin should be used in the case of multidrug resistant gram-positive isolates [9, 31]. Lately is noted increasing resistance for ofloxacin and ciprofloxacin; hereof, moxifloxacin and gatifloxacin are being used with more efficacy in managing bacterial keratitis [56].

Aminoglycosides are the second group of antibiotics that should be considered when treating BK. Aminoglycosides are represented by amikacin 0,3% topical eye drops (fortified amikacin eyedrops: 40 mg/ml), neomycin 0,5% eye ointment, gentamicin 0,3% topical eye drops (fortified gentamicin eye drops: 14 mg/ml (1.4%)), and tobramycin - 0,3% topical eye drops (fortified tobramycin eye drops: 14 mg/ml (1.4%)). Due to the broad spectrum of activity against gram-positive bacteria (excluding streptococci and pneumococci) and gram-negative bacteria, they are combined in the first line with fluoroquinolones. The mechanism of action of the fluoroquinolones is blocking of topoisomerase IV and DNA gyrase. The mechanism of action of aminoglycosides is to block protein synthesis at the ribosomal level. The combination of antibiotics from both groups is effective in the treatment of an unspecified etiological factor.

Other antibiotics that demonstrate a high therapeutic effectiveness in BK is vancomycin, which is used in severe infections. Fortified vancomycin 5% is very active against methicillin-resistant *Staphylococcus aureus* (MRSA). Whereas topical cefazolin 5% (fortified) is best appropriate for non-penicillinase-producing gram-positive bacteria [56].

The systemic antibiotics have indications in non-resolving progressive bacterial ulcers, especially with associated scleritis or endophthalmitis [57]. Fluoroquinolones, which demonstrate excellent penetration into ocular tissues when combined with intensive topical antibiotic treatment, are especially recommended.

7.2 Topical corticosteroid therapy

The use of additional adjuvant topical corticosteroid therapy remains still controversial [12, 58]. When the disease process is advanced and tissue necrosis occurs, or when inflammation is accompanied by intense cellular inflammatory infiltration into the cornea, weak steroids could be used. Topical corticosteroid therapy should be used with caution under constant clinical observation of the patient's involving eye because it may worsen the infection, local immunosuppression, corneal melting, and increased intraocular pressure [9, 58]. Topical corticosteroid therapy is used as an aim of suppression of inflammation to reduce corneal scarring, neovascularization, and vision loss. Hence, common or indiscriminate use of corticosteroids is inappropriate; however, it do not appear to increase the overall risk of failure or management of BK.

7.3 Other topical drugs therapy

Cycloplegics medications are commonly used as adjuvant drugs to relieve the pain, reduce ciliary spasm, and reduce cells and flare, as well as to prevent posterior synechiae formation that is often associated with iritis accompanying BK. They are indicated in cases with significant anterior chamber inflammation [12, 55, 56]. Antiglaucoma drugs are useful to control and reducing intraocular pressure by help drain the hypopyon by opening the trabecular meshwork and drainage channels, as well as to help in controlling trabeculitis secondary to the inflammatory process. A total of 0.5% timolol is commonly used. Two groups of topical drugs should be avoided, namely prostaglandin analogs and miotics because they exacerbate inflammation of the eye [12, 55, 56].

There should also be taken care of basic hygiene measures, which include careful removal of residual purulent secretion, which contains enzymes from decayed and endotoxins of dead bacteria, which makes it difficult for drugs to penetrate into the tissues. The moisturizing of the eye surface with the use of artificial tear preparations, that purpose is to restore disturbed homeostasis of the eye surface, as well as to help epithelial healing, reduce irritation, wash away debris and necrotic enzymes, and smoothen the ocular surface and cornea are also important.

7.4 Surgical treatment

Corneal cross-linking (CXL) is a relatively new option for anti-infective treatment, especially in cases of superficial bacterial keratitis, and is increasingly used as an additional adjuvant treatment, which has been confirmed in clinical trials [59–61]. The interaction of UV light and riboflavin damages the DNA and RNA of bacterial and viral pathogens and prevents their protein synthesis and replication, leading to the death of the microorganism [62]. Moreover, the cornea after CXL is more resistant to proteolytic enzymes produced by bacteria [63]. CXL, besides as adjuvant treatment for BK, can be also used as primary treatment in the early stages of infectious ulcerative keratitis. PACK-CXL (photoactivated chromophore for keratitis) is the procedure that uses of CXL besides the Dresden protocol for the treatment of infectious keratitis [60]. PACK-CXL, as an additional to the standard of care in cases of culture-proven bacterial keratitis, has a positive effect on the final visual acuity and time to resolution, compared with the standard-of-care treatment [64]. Recently studies reported that CXL therapy for IK patients with corneal thinning and/or including anterior part of the stroma is promising procedure [65].

There are several cases in which surgical interventions are indicated. The application of cyanoacrylate tissue adhesive is the first-line intervention for corneal perforation, providing a successful tectonic support for a short time, although requiring reapplication with a month after first application [66]. Depending on the cause of the perforation, indications for applications, and definition of success the success of this adhesive ranges between 29% and 86% [66].

Amniotic membrane has a great effect in acceleration corneal healing. Amniotic membrane transplantation (AMT) is an alternative therapeutic treatment option to cyanoacrylate glue application along with bandage contact lens (BCL) in the case of impending corneal perforation or corneal perforation [66, 67]. Although in the case of larger perforation (>2 mm), therapeutic keratoplasty should be performed.

Conjunctival flap (Gunderson flap) is another alternative treatment in the case of impending corneal perforation or corneal perforation if a donor cornea is unavailable. Conjunctival flap is considered as one of the oldest methods to treat corneal perforation when access to corneal graft is impossible [68]. In order to implement the accurate role of the conjunctival flap in treatment before keratoplasty in cases of BK there are needed extra studies. The technique relies on dissection of the upper conjunctiva, and a thin flap of the conjunctiva is covered over the cornea and sutured [69].

Therapeutic penetrating keratoplasty is used in the treatment of BK and is indicated when the disease progresses despite treatment, nonhealing corneal ulcers (above 2 weeks), descemetocele or perforation occurs, or keratitis does not respond to antimicrobial treatment [70]. Therapeutic penetrating keratoplasty helps eliminate the focus of infection and as a tectonic keratoplasty restores anatomical integrity in perforated corneal ulcers. During the procedure, it is advisable to remove all areas of infection and perform peripheral iridectomy because the pupil may be secclusio due to inflammatory membranes in its lumen. When exudates are present in the lens or there is a cataract, then the lens is removed. If the posterior capsule is tact, a thorough anterior vitrectomy is made. Clearing corneal margin of 0.5 mm from the diseased cornea is removed and put the graft is kept 0.5 mm larger than the host cornea. It is recommended to use single seams (9–0 or 10–0 nylon). After the procedure, topical antibiotics, cycloplegics, and topical steroids are used. Although the probability of graft survival is reduced in about a half, at 4 years post-intervention, in eyes with inflammation or with corticosteroid use at the time of graft, therapeutic penetrating keratoplasty remains the major intervention for the management of rapidly progressing severe infections and in large corneal perforations [67, 70]. When the visual acuity is poor, the cornea has scarred and healed and the infective foci have been eliminated after BK treatment penetrating keratoplasty (PKP) can be performed in order to restore the patient's vision. PKP is possible to conduct after 6 to 8 months of quieted after BK treatment [70].

7.5 Alternatives methods of treatment

In the literature based on animal studies showed that cryotherapy may have a possible advantageous result on BK involving the sclera. Although more studies about cryotherapy on the human cornea are still essential to answer for its efficacy and safety on human corneas [71, 72].

Mitomycin C (MMC) is an antimetabolite isolated from Streptomyces caespitosus. MMS has been successfully used in refractive surgery to reduce postoperative corneal haze and scaring due to its anti-fibroblast activity [73]. In one research, authors found that MMS has a broad-spectrum antimicrobial activity against a broad range of bacteria, including *E. coli*, *S. aureus*, and *P. aeruginosa* [74]. However, further studies are required to evaluate the effect of MMC on human corneas in BK because above mentioned results from laboratory studies are limited. While the inflammation process (i.e., an acute infection) and inflammatory cells (such as keratocytes, fibroblasts) produce enzymes: collagenases and matrix metalloproteinases (MMPs) that are involved in protein degradation and keratolysis. Anti-collagenases are promising adjuvant option in treatment BK though there are no high-quality randomized controlled trials in humans to help clinicians in the use of doxycycline for the corneal ulceration treatment, although its widespread use among corneal specialists [75–77].

Antimicrobial photodynamic therapy is another new approach for IK treatment based on three agents: oxygen, light radiation, and photosensitizer. Photodynamic therapy has proved as an effective therapy against infectious agents it does not present selective pressure on resistance development by both gram-positive and gram-negative bacteria. Thus, this new treatment option has an unusual potential for treatment of BK cases that have not achieved a good response after traditional antibiotic therapy [78].

In the newest reports, the bacteriophage therapy is growing as an effective alternative to treat ocular infections. A variety of nanotechnology-based formulations, such as nanoemulsions, liposomes, polymeric nanoparticles, dendrimers, and nanofibres, have been recently reported to be effective results in bacteria resistance to antibiotics. There are bacteriophage-based nanoformulation techniques for the successful treatment of ocular infections caused by multidrug-resistant S. aureus and other bacteria [79].

8. Conclusions

Corneal opacity represents the fifth leading cause of blindness globally, with infectious keratitis being the main culprit. Bacterial keratitis is a severe condition of the eyes that could have a burden impact on human health in both developed and developing countries. Understanding of the major risk factors for BK particularly CL wear, trauma, ocular surface diseases, and postocular surgery will simplify a more effective public health intervention to modify and reduce the risk of BK. Early and prompt medical treatment is needed to avoid complications. The vision-threatening bacterial ulcers, if treated on time, can have an excellent visual effect. In the past few decades, it has been observed the increased rate of antimicrobial resistance (AMR) in ocular infection in several countries highlights the need for reasonable use of antibiotics. It should be a tighter control of OTC antibiotics and development of new therapeutic strategies. Improvement in the diagnostic efficiency of microbiological investigations of BK with emerging new technologies will allow for fast and proper diagnosis and could also provide a better guidance on the appropriate use of antimicrobial therapy in the future, eventually reducing the risk of AMR. The prognosis of BK is governed by a multiplicity of factors. The good prognosis for BK is in the case of bacterial ulcer located in the superficial corneal layers (anterior one-third of the stroma), as well as a result of a good compliance between doctor and patient and regular follow-up, and regular use of medications. Involvement of sclera or endophthalmitis, ulcer involving more than two-thirds of stroma, located in the visual axis, stromal melt, and corneal thinning exacerbate much more the prognosis. New approaches for the treatment of bacterial keratitis are necessary to outcome the increasing antibiotic resistance.

Conflict of interest

The authors declare no conflict of interest.

Acronyms and abbreviations

BK	bacterial keratitis
IK	infectious keratitis
MK	microbial keratitis
OSD	ocular surface disease
CL	contact lens
AMR	antimicrobial resistance
PCR test	polymerase chain reaction test
IVCM	*in vivo* confocal microscopy
CXL	corneal cross-linking
PACK-CXL	photoactivated chromophore for keratitis
PKP	penetrating keratoplasty
AMT	amniotic membrane transplantation
MMC	mitomycin C
MMPs	matrix metalloproteinases

Author details

Edyta Chlasta-Twardzik[1*] and Anna Nowińska[2]

1 Ophthalmology Department, Railway Hospital, Katowice, Poland

2 Clinical Department of Ophthalmology, Faculty of Medical Sciences in Zabrze, Medical University of Silesia, Katowice, Poland

*Address all correspondence to: edyta.chlasta@gmail.com

References

[1] Flaxman SR, Bourne RRA, Resnikoff S, Ackland P, Braithwaite T, Cicinelli MV, et al. Global causes of blindness and distance vision impairment 1990-2020: A systematic review and meta-analysis. The Lancet Global Health. 2017;**5**:e1221-e1e34

[2] Whitcher JP, Srinivasan M, Upadhyay MP. Corneal blindness: A global perspective. Bulletin of the World Health Organization. 2001;**79**:214-221

[3] Shivangi C, Pravin Tidake. A review of corneal blindness: Causes and management; Cureus. Oct 2022;**14**(10):e30097. Available from: https://www.who.int/news-room/fact-sheets/detail/trachoma [Accessed: October 9, 2022]

[4] Durand ML, Barshak MB, Chodosh J. Infectious keratitis in 2021. Journal of the American Medical Association. 2021;**326**(13):1319-1320

[5] Shah A, Sachdev A, Coggon D. Geographic variations in microbial keratitis: An analysis of the peer-reviewed literature. The British Journal of Ophthalmology. 2011;**95**:762-767

[6] Christy J, Gurnani B, Kaur K, Moutappa F. Contact lens warpage: Lost but found. Indian Journal of Ophthalmology. 2020;**68**(8):1662

[7] Bollag WB, Olala LO, Xie D, Lu X, Qin H, Choudhary V, et al. Dioleoylphosphatidylglycerol accelerates corneal epithelial wound healing. Investigative Ophthalmology and Visual Science. 2020;**61**:29. DOI: 10.1167/iovs.61.3.29

[8] Ung L, Bispo PJM, Shanbhag SS, Gilmore MS, Chodosh J. The persistent dilemma of microbial keratitis: Global burden, diagnosis, and antimicrobial resistance. Survey of Ophthalmology. 2019;**64**:255-271

[9] Lin A, Rhee MK, Akpek EK, et al. Bacterial keratitis preferred practice pattern®. Ophthalmology. 2019;**126**(1):P1-P55

[10] Tjia KF, van Putten JP, Pels E, Zanen HC. The interaction between Neisseria gonorrhoeae and the human cornea in organ culture. An electron microscopic study. Graefe's Archive for Clinical and Experimental Ophthalmology. 1988;**226**(4):341-345

[11] Khoo P, Cabrera-Aguas MP, Nguyen V, Lahra MM, Watson SL. Microbial keratitis in Sydney, Australia: Risk factors, patient outcomes, and seasonal variation. Graefe's Archive for Clinical and Experimental Ophthalmology. 2020;**258**(8):1745-1755

[12] Austin A, Lietman T, Rose-Nussbaumer J. Update on the management of infectious keratitis. Ophthalmology. 2017;**124**(11):1678-1689

[13] Stapleton F. Contact lens-related corneal infection in Australia. Clinical & Experimental Optometry. 2020;**103**:408-417

[14] Young AL, Leung KS, Tsim N, Hui M, Jhanji V. Risk factors, microbiological profile, and treatment outcomes of pediatric microbial keratitis in a tertiary care hospital in Hong Kong. American Journal of Ophthalmology. 2013;**156**(5):1040-1044.e2

[15] Jin H, Parker WT, Law NW, Clarke CL, Gisseman JD, Pflugfelder SC, et al. Evolving risk factors and antibiotic

sensitivity patterns for microbial keratitis at a large county hospital. The British Journal of Ophthalmology. 2017;**101**(11):1483-1487

[16] Keay L, Edwards K, Naduvilath T, Taylor HR, Snibson GR, Forde K, et al. Microbial keratitis predisposing factors and morbidity. Ophthalmology. 2006;**113**(1):109-116

[17] Ting DSJ, Ho CS, Cairns J, Elsahn A, Al-Aqaba M, Boswell T, et al. 12-year analysis of incidence, microbiological profiles and in vitro antimicrobial susceptibility of infectious keratitis: The Nottingham infectious keratitis study. The British Journal of Ophthalmology. Mar 2021;**105**(3):328-333. DOI: 10.1136/bjophthalmol-2020-316128

[18] Tavassoli S, Nayar G, Darcy K, Grzeda M, Luck J, Williams OM, et al. An 11-year analysis of microbial keratitis in the south west of England using brain-heart infusion broth. Eye (London, England). 2019;**33**:1619-1625

[19] Politis M, Wajnsztajn D, Rosin B, Block C, Solomon A. Trends of bacterial keratitis culture isolates in Jerusalem; a 13-years analysis. PLoS One. 2016;**11**:e0165223

[20] Tam ALC, Côté E, Saldanha M, Lichtinger A, Slomovic AR. Bacterial keratitis in Toronto: A 16-year review of the microorganisms isolated and the resistance patterns observed. Cornea. 2017;**36**:1528-1534

[21] Hernandez-Camarena JC, Graue-Hernandez EO, Ortiz-Casas M, Ramirez-Miranda A, Navas A, Pedro-Aguilar L, et al. Trends in microbiological and antibiotic sensitivity patterns in infectious keratitis: 10-year experience in Mexico City. Cornea. 2015;**34**:778-785

[22] Cabrera-Aguas M, Khoo P, George CRR, Lahra MM, Watson S. Antimicrobial resistance trends in bacterial keratitis over 5 years in Sydney, Australia. Clinical & Experimental Ophthalmology. 2019;**48**:183-191

[23] Upadhyay MP, Karmacharya PC, Koirala S, Shah DN, Shakya S, Shrestha JK, et al. The Bhaktapur eye study: Ocular trauma and antibiotic prophylaxis for the prevention of corneal ulceration in Nepal. The British Journal of Ophthalmology. 2001;**85**(4):388-392

[24] Bharathi MJ, Ramakrishnan R, Meenakshi R, Padmavathy S, Shivakumar C, Srinivasan M. Microbial keratitis in South India: Influence of risk factors, climate, and geographical variation. Ophthalmic Epidemiology. 2007;**14**(2):61-69

[25] Alipour F, Khaheshi S, Soleimanzadeh M, Heidarzadeh S, Heydarzadeh S. Contact lens-related complications: A review. Journal of Ophthalmic & Vision Research. 2017;**12**(2):193-204

[26] Fleiszig SMJ, Kroken AR, Nieto V, Grosser MR, Wan SJ, Metruccio MME, et al. Contact lens-related corneal infection: Intrinsic resistance and its compromise. Progress in Retinal and Eye Research. 2020;**76**:100804

[27] Acharya M, Farooqui JH, Jain S, Mathur U. Pearls and paradigms in infective keratitis. Romanian Journal of Ophthalmology. 2019;**63**(2):119-127

[28] Al-Mujaini A, Al-Kharusi N, Thakral A, Wali UK. Bacterial keratitis: Perspective on epidemiology, clinico-pathogenesis, diagnosis and treatment. Sultan Qaboos University Medical Journal. 2009;**9**(2):184-195

[29] Tabbara KF, El-Asrar AMA, Khairallah M. Ocular Infections: Infectious Keratitis. Springer; 2014

[30] Dini LA, Cockinos C, Frean JA, Niszl IA, Markus MB. Unusual case of Acanthamoeba polyphaga and Pseudomonas aeruginosa keratitis in a contact lens wearer from Gauteng, South Africa. Journal of Clinical Microbiology. 2000;**38**(2):826-829

[31] Cabrera-Aguas M, Khoo P, Watson SL. Infectious keratitis: A review; Clinical & Experimental Ophthalmology. Jul 2022;**50**(5):543-562

[32] Garg P, Roy A. Clinical work-up of corneal ulcers. In: Das S, Jhanji V, editors. Infections of the Cornea and Conjunctiva. Springer Singapore; 2021. pp. 75-84

[33] Leck A. Taking a corneal scrape and making a diagnosis. Community Eye Health. 2009;**22**(71):42-43

[34] Ngo J, Khoo P, Watson SL. Improving the efficiency and the technique of the corneal scrape procedure via an evidence based instructional video at a quaternary referral eye hospital. Current Eye Research. 2020;**45**(5):529-534

[35] Bonnet M, Lagier JC, Raoult D, Khelaifia S. Bacterial culture through selective and non-selective conditions: The evolution of culture media in clinical microbiology. New Microbes New Infections. 2020;**34**:100622

[36] Ting DSJ, Ho CS, Cairns J, et al. 12-year analysis of incidence, microbiological profiles and in vitro antimicrobial susceptibility of infectious keratitis: The Nottingham infectious keratitis study. The British Journal of Ophthalmology. 2021;**105**(3):328-333

[37] Green M, Carnt N, Apel A, et al. Queensland microbial keratitis database: 2005-2015. The British Journal of Ophthalmology. 2019;**103**(10):1481-1486

[38] Watson SL, Gatus BJ, Cabrera-Aguas M, et al. Bacterial ocular surveillance system (BOSS) Sydney, Australia 2017-2018. Communicable Diseases Intelligence. 2020:25-44. DOI: 10.33321/cdi.2020.44.86

[39] Das S, Samantaray R, Mallick A, Sahu SK, Sharma S. Types of organisms and in-vitro susceptibility of bacterial isolates from patients with microbial keratitis: A trend analysis of 8 years. Indian Journal of Ophthalmology. 2019;**67**(1):49-53

[40] Khor HG, Cho I, Lee KRCK, Chieng LL. Spectrum of microbial keratitis encountered in the tropics. Eye & Contact Lens. 2020;**46**(1):17-23

[41] Soleimani M, Tabatabaei SA, Masoumi A, et al. Infectious keratitis: Trends in microbiological and antibiotic sensitivity patterns. Eye (London, England). 2021;**35**(11):3110-3115

[42] de Luiza Manhezi Shin O, Tatiana T, Juliana Mika K, et al. Research Square. 2021.

[43] Alexandrakis G, Haimovici R, Miller D, Alfonso EC. Corneal biopsy in the management of progressive microbial keratitis. American Journal of Ophthalmology. 2000;**129**(5):571-576

[44] Everts RJ, Barnett T, Lahood BR. The utility of routine conjunctival swabs in management of conjunctivitis. The New Zealand Medical Journal. 2011;**124**(1328):64-71

[45] Sridhar MS, Sharma S, Gopinathan U, Rao GN. Anterior chamber tap: Diagnostic and therapeutic indications in the management of ocular infections. Cornea. 2002;**21**(7):718-722

[46] Das S, Sheorey H, Taylor HR, Vajpayee RB. Association between cultures of contact lens and corneal scraping in contact lens related microbial

keratitis. Archives of Ophthalmology. 2007;**125**(9):1182-1185

[47] Willcox MDP. Characterization of the normal microbiota of the ocular surface. Experimental Eye Research. 2013;**117**:99-105

[48] Hoffman JJ, Dart JKG, De SK, et al. Comparison of culture, confocal microscopy and PCR in routine hospital use for microbial keratitis diagnosis. Eye. 2022;**36**:2172-2178. DOI: 10.1038/s41433-021-01812-7

[49] Robaei D, Chan UT, Khoo P, et al. Corneal biopsy for diagnosis of recalcitrant microbial keratitis. Graefe's Archive for Clinical and Experimental Ophthalmology. 2018;**256**(8):1527-1533

[50] Somerville TF, Corless CE, Sueke H, Neal T, Kaye SB. 16S ribosomal RNA PCR versus conventional diagnostic culture in the investigation of suspected bacterial keratitis. Translational Vision Science & Technology. 2020;**9**(13):2

[51] Liu HY, Hopping GC, Vaidyanathan U, Ronquillo YC, Hoopes PC, Moshirfar M. Polymerase chain reaction and its application in the diagnosis of infectious keratitis. Medical Hypothesis, Discovery & Innovation Ophthalmology Journal. 2019;**8**(3):152-155

[52] Sahay P, Goel S, Nagpal R, et al. Infectious keratitis caused by rare and emerging micro-organisms. Current Eye Research. 2020;**45**(7):761-773

[53] Wang YE, Tepelus TC, Vickers LA, Baghdasaryan E, Gui W, Huang P, et al. Role of in vivo confocal microscopy in the diagnosis of infectious keratitis. International Ophthalmology. 2019;**39**:2865-2874

[54] Kumar RL, Cruzat A, Hamrah P. Current state of in vivo confocal microscopy in management of microbial keratitis. Seminars in Ophthalmology. 2010;**25**:166-170

[55] Solanki S, Rathi M, Khanduja S, Dhull CS, Sachdeva S, Phogat J. Recent trends: Medical management of infectious keratitis. Oman Journal of Ophthalmology. 2015;**8**(2):83-85

[56] Gokhale NS. Medical management approach to infectious keratitis. Indian Journal of Ophthalmology. 2008;**56**(3):215-220

[57] Daniell M. Overview: Initial antimicrobial therapy for microbial keratitis. The British Journal of Ophthalmology. 2003;**87**(9):1172-1174

[58] Khoo P, Cabrera-Aguas M, Watson SL. Topical steroids as adjunctive therapy for bacterial keratitis: Evidence from a retrospective case series of 313 cases. Asia-Pacific Journal of Ophthalmology (Philadelphia, PA.). 2020;**9**(5):398-403

[59] Makdoumi K, Mortensen J, Crafoord S. Infectious keratitis treated with corneal crosslinking. Cornea. 2010;**29**:1353-1358

[60] Said DG, Elalfy MS, Gatzioufas Z, et al. Collagen cross-linking with photoactivated riboflavin (PACK-CXL) for the treatment of advanced infectious keratitis with corneal melting. Ophthalmology. 2014;**121**:1377-1382

[61] Ting DSJ, Henein C, Said DG, Dua HS. Effectiveness of adjuvant photoactivated chromophore corneal collagen cross-linking versus standard antimicrobial treatment for infectious keratitis: A systematic review protocol. JBI Database of Systematic Reviews and Implementation Reports. Jan 2020;**18**(1):194-199

[62] Martins SA, Combs JC, Noguera G, et al. Antimicrobial efficacy of

riboflavin/UVA combination (365 nm) in vitro for bacterial and fungal isolates: A potential new treatment for infectious keratitis. Investigative Ophthalmology & Visual Science. 2008;**49**:3402-3408

[63] Spoerl E, Wollensak G, Seiler T. Increased resistance of crosslinked cornea against enzymatic digestion. Current Eye Research. 2004;**29**:35-40

[64] Achiron A, Elhaddad O, Regev T, Krakauer Y, Tsumi E, Hafezi F, et al. PACK cross-linking as adjuvant therapy improves clinical outcomes in culture-confirmed bacterial keratitis. Cornea. 2022;**41**(9):1069-1073

[65] Bonzano C, Di Zazzo A, Barabino S, Coco G, Traverso CE. Collagen cross-linking in the management of microbial keratitis. Ocular Immunology and Inflammation. 2019;**27**:507-512

[66] Yin J, Singh RB, Al Karmi R, et al. Outcomes of cyanoacrylate tissue adhesive application in corneal thinning and perforation. Cornea. 2019;**38**(6):668-673

[67] Ung L, Chodosh J. Foundational concepts in the biology of bacterial keratitis. Experimental Eye Research. 2021;**209**:108647

[68] Gundersen T. Conjunctival flaps in the treatment of corneal disease with reference to a new technique of application. A.M.A. Archives of Ophthalmology. 1958;**60**:880-888

[69] Zemba M, Stamate AC, Tataru CP, Branisteanu DC, Balta F. Conjunctival flap surgery in the management of ocular surface disease (review). Experimental and Therapeutic Medicine. 2020;**20**(4):3412-3416

[70] Gurnani B, Christy J, Narayana S, Rajkumar P, Kaur K, Gubert J. Retrospective multifactorial analysis of Pythium keratitis and review of literature. Indian Journal of Ophthalmology. 2021;**69**(5):1095-1101

[71] Alpren TV, Hyndiuk RA, Davis SD, Sarff LD. Cryotherapy for experimental pseudomonas keratitis. Archives of Ophthalmology (Chicago, ILL: 1960). 1979;**97**:711-714

[72] Eiferman RA. Cryotherapy of Pseudonomas keratitis and scleritis. Archives of Ophthalmology. 1979;**97**:1637-1639

[73] Carones F, Vigo L, Scandola E, Vacchini L. Evaluation of the prophylactic use of mitomycin-C to inhibit haze formation after photorefractive keratectomy. Journal of Cataract and Refractive Surgery. 2002;**28**:2088-2095

[74] Kwan BW, Chowdhury N, Wood TK. Combatting bacterial infections by killing persister cells with mitomycin C. Environmental Microbiology. 2015;**17**:4406-4414

[75] Burns FR, Stack MS, Gray RD, Paterson CA. Inhibition of purified collagenase from alkali-burned rabbit corneas. Investigative Ophthalmology & Visual Science. 1989;**30**(7):1569-1575

[76] Golub LM, Sorsa T, Lee HM, et al. Doxycycline inhibits neutrophil (PMN)-type matrix metalloproteinases in human adult periodontitis gingiva. Journal of Clinical Periodontology. Feb 1995;**22**(2):100-109

[77] Dursun D, Kim MC, Solomon A, Pflugfelder SC. Treatment of recalcitrant recurrent corneal erosions with inhibitors of matrix metalloproteinase-9, doxycycline and corticosteroids. American Journal of Ophthalmology. 2001;**132**(1):8-13

[78] de Paiva ACM, Ferreira MDC, da Fonseca AS. Photodynamic therapy

for treatment of bacterial keratitis. Photodiagnosis and Photodynamic Therapy. 2022;**37**:102717

[79] Patil R, Dehari D, Chaudhuri A, Kumar DN, Kumar D, Singh S, et al. Recent advancements in nanotechnology-based bacteriophage delivery strategies against bacterial ocular infections. Microbiological Research. 2023;**273**:127413

Chapter 2

Infectious Keratitis after Surgery

Alberto Haber Olguin, Guillermo Raúl Vera Duarte and Luis Antonio García Padilla

Abstract

Although infectious keratitis after refractive surgery is rare, it is of great importance due to its great devastating power. The most important etiology of infectious keratitis after refractive surgery is: *Staphylococcus epidermidis*. The risk factors associated with the development of infectious keratitis are divided into: pre-surgical, intra-surgical and post-surgical. The time of onset of symptoms after refractive surgery is one of the most important antecedents associated with the causative microorganism. Less than 7 days is considered "early onset". After 7 days of "late onset." The initiation of empirical treatment is recommended in the case of early onset of symptoms with 4th generation fluoroquinolone alternated with fortified cefazolin. In the case of late onset (more than 7 days after surgery), start with 4th generation fluoroquinolone alternating with Amikacin as well as oral doxycycline. At the end of the surgery, it is recommended to apply a drop of moxifloxacin. Regarding post-surgical measures, the time of contact lens use should be limited, avoid contaminated environments and administer antibiotics for a period of 7–10 days, or until the epithelial defect has been completely resolved.

Keywords: refractive surgery, LASIK, PRK, SMILE, infectious keratitis, infectious keratitis etiology, differential diagnosis, infectious keratitis, infectious keratitis treatment

1. Introduction

Among the complications after refractive surgery is keratitis, of which there are infectious and non-infectious types. Non-infectious keratitis is the most frequent and generally has the best prognosis. As for infectious infiltrative keratitis, it is a relatively uncommon clinical entity, although a very feared one.

The corneal defense mechanisms against infections are varied and generally effective; within these mechanisms are the following [1, 2]:

- The constant flow of tears that is produced in the conjunctiva and distributed by the eyelid all over the surface of the cornea minimizes the accumulation of detritus.

- The corneal epithelium is a semipermeable physical barrier in which the rapid turnover of cells, their desquamation, and the tear film make bacterial adhesion difficult.

- The corneal temperature is lower than that of the rest of the body, thus hampering bacterial replication.
- The tear contains lysozymes, i.e., lactoferrins which are enzymes that limit bacterial growth.

All these mechanisms, however, can become impaired in cases of trauma, burns, alterations of the ocular surface, and also in some cases of refractive surgery.

Photoablative refractive surgery, either laser in situ keratomileusis (LASIK) or surface surgery (PRK), makes the cornea more liable to infections. Although infectious keratitis is a rare complication, it can also be devastating if adequate and timely measures are not taken [2]. As for the novel technique of small incision lenticule extraction (SMILE), only a few cases of infectious keratitis have been described so far [3–5].

2. Etiology

Even during refractive surgery there may be contamination by bacteria in the corneal stroma in up to 24% of cases. These bacteria are mostly of Gram-positive type, in most cases, *Staphylococcus epidermidis*, which does not necessarily manifest as infectious keratitis due to stromal defense mechanisms [6]. The causative agents fall within the same spectrum across the different surgical techniques. Atypical mycobacterial keratitis related to inadequate sterilization has also been described, including superficial punctate keratitis, contact lens use, and other history of previous refractive surgery or touch-ups, particularly radial keratotomy [7, 8].

Currently, the most frequently related agents are Gram-positive cocci [8, 9]. Although less frequently, other possible causative agents have been reported, namely, additional Gram-positive bacteria such as *Nocardia spp* and *Corynebacterium spp*, Gram-negative bacteria such as *Pseudomonas aeruginosa* and *Serratia*, fungi, *Acanthamoeba*, and even polymicrobial infections. Also, among the most common causative agents of viral infections are adenovirus [10–13].

3. Risk factors

The following have been identified as the main predisposing factors for infection: disruption of the barrier function of the corneal epithelium, use of bandage contact lenses and topical corticosteroids, history of blepharitis, previous corneal surgery, contamination during surgery, dry eye, lack of perioperative antibiotics, and herpes simplex virus (HSV) infection [14, 15]. The use of contaminated surgical instruments, the surgeon's hands, the presence of infectious agents on the ocular surface, and environmental conditions could also be associated with contamination and hence with the development of corneal infections [16].

Several factors inherent in the procedure explain the increased risk of infection after a photorefractive keratectomy (PRK) compared with other techniques. Among them, the defect in the epithelium caused during surgery, and the time of about 4 days for its regeneration, entails a loss of the protective function of the corneal epithelium and may create an area prone to adhesion and reproduction of microorganisms. Other factors are the use of therapeutic contact lenses, which are routinely used after surgery, and the use of topical corticosteroids [15, 17].

Preoperative	Dry eye
	Blepharitis, Meibomian gland dysfunction
Intraoperative	Inadequate sterilization
	PRK > LASIK
	Use of contact lenses
	Face masks
Postoperative	Use of contact lenses
	Epithelial defect
	Iadequate postoperative follow-up
	Poor postoperative hygiene
	Healthcare workers
	Face masks

Table 1.
Risk factors associated with infectious keratitis.

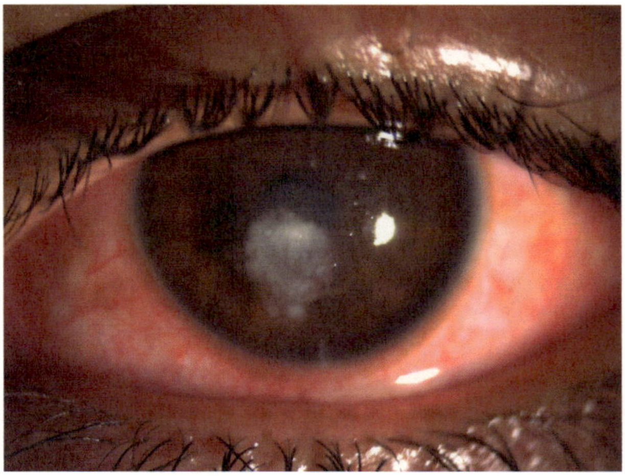

Figure 1.
Slit-lamp microscopy image of the patient's right eye showing a central infectious infiltrate.

In addition, a recent retrospective study has linked the use of face masks in the previous COVID-19 pandemic with a slight increase in the incidence of infectious keratitis in patients undergoing refractive surgery [18]. Another risk factor to be considered is the possible link with methyl-resistant infectious agents [18, 19] (**Table 1** and **Figure 1**).

4. Epidemiology

The incidence of infectious keratitis following refractive surgery varies according to different studies. A major review reported a frequency of 1 in 1000 for PRK, and 1 in 5000 for LASIK [13, 20]. The higher incidence of infectious keratitis for PKR than for LASIK is evident in multiple studies [15, 19]. On the other hand, there is little evidence and few studies yet on the frequency and treatment of infectious keratitis after SMILE [3, 4, 21].

5. Diagnosis

The clinical presentation of an infection after refractive surgery comprises decreased visual acuity, secretion, pain, epithelial defect, flap edema, reaction in anterior chamber, ciliary injection, and lacrimation. The signs and symptoms are much more varied in the case of infections by bacteria than by fungi and mycobacteria, where the symptoms can be at first frankly discreet [22].

The time of symptom onset after refractive surgery is one of the most important antecedents associated with the causative microorganism. If the symptoms begin within 7 days after the procedure (early onset), it is more likely that the infection is caused by Gram-positive bacteria or mycobacteria. If the symptoms appear after 7 days of the procedure (late onset) there is a greater likelihood that the causative agent is a mycobacterium, a fungus, Gram-positive bacteria or an *Acanthamoeba* [22–25]. As for *Acanthamoeba* keratitis, it is considered of late-onset and is often not directly related to surgical intervention, but to either the incorrect use of contact lenses or contaminated liquids. It could also occur due to a previous infection. For instance, if surgical interventions such as LASIK are performed on the cornea, intrastromal cysts could be reactivated [26, 27].

For several reasons, bacterial keratitis after refractive surgery presents some variants with respect to infectious infiltrative keratitis not associated with photoablation procedures. In the case of LASIK, it is during the procedure that we take the microorganism to the depth of the corneal stroma and then cover it with the flap. Consequently, an ulcer as such is not observed but rather an abscess below the flap or on the ablated stroma in the case of PRK may appear [28].

6. Differential diagnosis

The clinical presentation of infectious keratitis is not usually easy to identify, the main differential diagnoses are the following:

- Inflammatory infiltrates: These are dense clusters of inflammatory cells that manifest as an opacity generally less than 1 mm in diameter and poorly defined limits. The treatment is based on steroidal anti-inflammatories, which are contraindicated in presence of infection. They can appear 24–48 h after refractive surgery and do not usually show the inflammatory features of bacterial keratitis [6, 10].

- Diffuse lamellar keratitis: It is an inflammatory condition that begins 24–48 h after refractive surgery. It looks as a diffuse opacity at the interface of the lamella with a morphology similar to desert sands (it is commonly known as Sahara sands), i.e., there are no dense clusters as in the case of inflammatory infiltrates, especially in the initial stages. Its treatment is based on steroidal anti-inflammatories, which are also contraindicated if there is infection. The rest of the eyeball is not usually involved, as it does not show ciliary injection, cellularity, and flare in the anterior chamber, which are usually present in infectious processes [29, 30].

- Interface fluid syndrome (IFS) or PISK (Pressure-Induced Stromal Keratopathy). It is a localized inflammation, showing fluid in the interface area or a diffuse haze between the interface area and the inner layer of the corneal tissue. It occurs due to increased intraocular pressure (IOP) as a response to corticosteroid

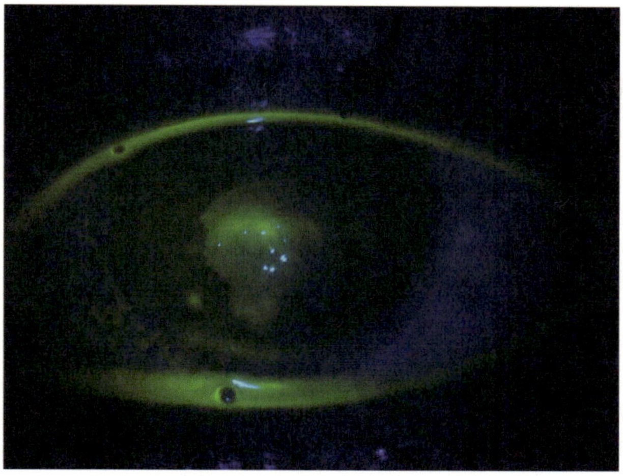

Figure 2.
Slit-lamp microscopy of the same patient's right eye showing corneal surface with fluorescein staining, showing the central epithelial defect.

treatment during the early postoperative phase (between 10 and 20 days). Cases have been reported even up to 10 years after surgery [31–33]. Measuring IOP increase can be difficult using Goldmann tonometry in the center of the cornea, so it is best doing it in the peripheral part of the cornea. This condition is managed using topical medications to reduce eye pressure. Contrary to most other complications, use of corticosteroids is not recommended; therefore, it is important to have an accurate differential diagnosis [34].

- Epithelial growth at the interface. It is caused by the proliferation of epithelial cells at the interface. It is whitish in appearance, painless, without inflammatory reaction, confined to the edge of the flap, and of later presentation. However, it can generate irregular astigmatism and decreased vision if the visual axis is compromised (**Figures 1** and **2**).

7. Treatment

Once the suspicion of infectious keratitis has been established, what follows is to lift the flap in the case of LASIK for taking cultures and washing with antibiotics. Some studies have shown that patients in whom this procedure is performed before 3 days after onset of symptoms have a better final visual capacity than those in whom this maneuver takes longer to be done [9, 22, 28].

During scraping, smears for Gram, Lowenstein-Jensen, and Middlebrook stains should be taken [30]. The culture should include media such as blood agar, chocolate, Sabouraud, and thioglycolate, with special emphasis on culture in special media such as Lowenstein-Jensen and Middlebrook in the event that the infection has appeared 7 days or more after surgery, considering atypical bacteria [30]. Culture results reveal that Gram-positive bacteria are the most common organisms present [8].

After taking the culture, it is recommended to wash the interface with fortified vancomycin 50 mg/ml in cases of early onset, and fortified amikacin 35 mg/ml in cases of late onset [30].

In most cases, the cause of the infection is difficult to determine. Among predisposing factor are the history of corneal surgery, excessive intraoperative manipulation, intraoperative contamination, and persistent postoperative epithelial defects of the cornea [7, 35, 36].

The start of empirical treatment is recommended in the case of early symptom onset with fourth-generation fluoroquinolone (after impregnation each 5 min for 30 min) alternated with fortified cefazolin 50 mg/ml every 30 min. In the case of patients who work in hospitals or who have been exposed to hospital environments, cefazolin should be replaced with fortified vancomycin 50 mg/ml due to the risk of methicillin-resistant *Staphylococcus aureus* (MRSA) [30].

In the case of late symptom onset (more than 7 days after surgery), treatment is started with fourth-generation fluoroquinolone (after impregnation) every 30 min, alternating with amikacin 35 mg/ml as well as doxycycline orally 100 mg 2 times a day [30].

Once the empirical treatment is commenced, the result of the stains and culture is expected. The stains are a useful guide, although their specificity and sensitivity may vary depending on the reported microorganism. The positive report of a stain for Gram-positive bacteria has a high sensitivity and a very low specificity, since these bacteria can be present on the ocular surface as normal flora. On the other hand, Gram-negative bacilli have a much higher sensitivity and specificity, and without waiting for culture results we can modify the empirical treatment initiated by replacing cefazolin or vancomycin with fortified ceftazidime [30].

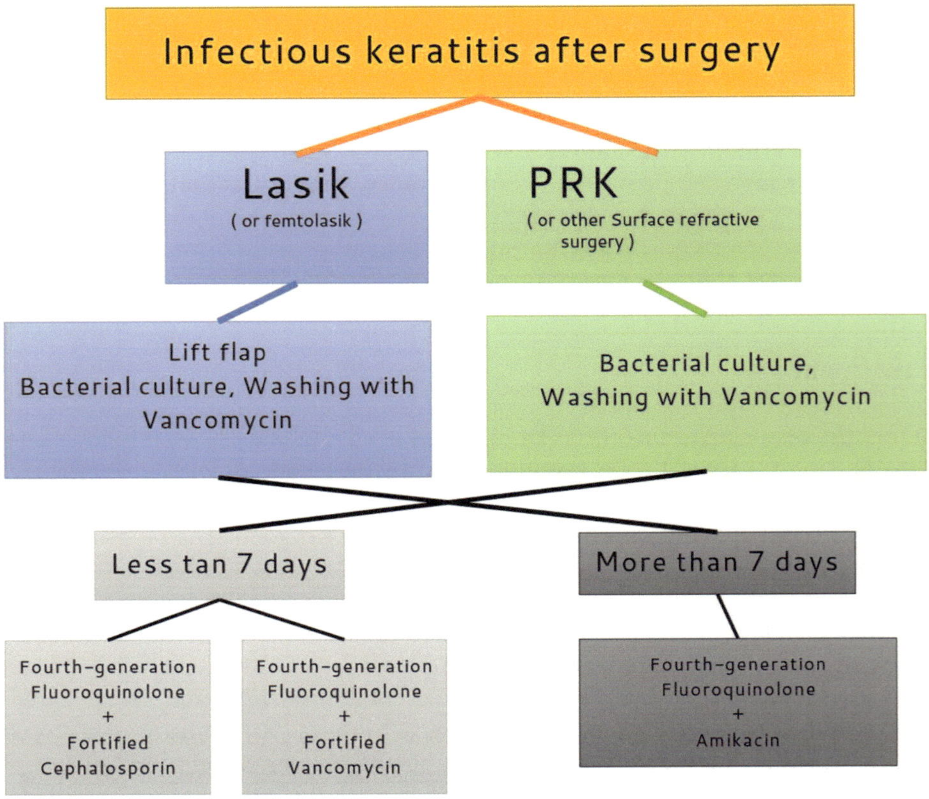

Figure 3.
Treatment nomogram.

Currently, new treatment modalities have emerged, such as corneal crosslinking, which is an alternative in cases where conventional medical treatment is not sufficient [3, 37]. Corneal crosslinking is highly recommended in patients who have undergone surgery with the SMILE technique [19]. As for antibiotic use, fourth-generation fluoroquinolones are not only a valuable tool in treatment, but are also useful for the prophylaxis of both lamellar and surface refractive procedures, showing superiority in comparison with other antibiotics, such as tobramycin (**Figure 3**) [17].

8. Prognosis

The prognosis of infectious keratitis is usually good. The best corrected visual acuity, 20/20 or better, is seen in 37% of cases, 20/40 or better in 76.5% of cases, and worse than 20/40 in 23.5% of cases [7]. Some important factors influencing visual prognosis are early diagnosis, removal of the contact lens, and early initiation of treatment with reinforced broad-spectrum antibiotics. However, it is not a complication that should be taken lightly; the literature reports flap amputations, perforations, keratoplasties, *acanthamoeba* infections, endophthalmitis, and even enucleation.

9. Prophylaxis

Among the prophylactic measures prior to surgery are the detection of alterations in the eyelids, blepharitis, and anomalies on the ocular surface. During the procedure, appropriate intraoperative measures must be taken, such as correct performance of asepsis, antisepsis, and proper sterilization of the instruments. Any debris present at the flap interface should be removed, as well as any textile material or tab. At the end of surgery, it is recommended to apply one drop of moxifloxacin 5 mg/ml. Regarding post-surgical measures, the time spent wearing contact lenses should be limited, contaminated environments should be avoided, and antibiotics should be administered for a period of 7–10 days, or until the epithelial defect has completely resolved [38].

10. Conclusion

An infection following refractive surgery is considered a potentially devastating complication, which could occur even months after surgery. Antibiotic prophylaxis is thus recommended to provide broad-spectrum coverage with focus on Gram-positive bacteria.

Author details

Alberto Haber Olguin*, Guillermo Raúl Vera Duarte and Luis Antonio García Padilla
Cornea and Refractive Surgery, Ophthalmology Institute "Conde de Valenciana" Foundation, Mexico Federal District, Mexico

*Address all correspondence to: doctorhaber@gmail.com

References

[1] Toda I. LASIK and the ocular surface. Cornea. 2008;**27**(Suppl. 1):S70-S76

[2] Rosman M, Chua WH, Tseng PSF, Wee TL, Chan WK. Diffuse lamellar keratitis after laser in situ keratomileusis associated with surgical marker pens. Journal of Cataract and Refractive Surgery. 2008;**34**(6):974-979

[3] Chan TCY, Chow VWS, Jhanji V. Collagen cross-linking with photoactivated riboflavin (PACK-CXL) for bacterial keratitis after small incision lenticule extraction (SMILE). Journal of Refractive Surgery Thorofare NJ 1995. 2007;**33**(4):278-280

[4] Chehaibou I, Sandali O, Ameline B, Bouheraoua N, Borderie V, Laroche L. Bilateral infectious keratitis after small-incision lenticule extraction. Journal of Cataract and Refractive Surgery. 2016;**42**(4):626-630

[5] Ivarsen A, Asp S, Hjortdal J. Safety and complications of more than 1500 small-incision lenticule extraction procedures. Ophthalmology. 2014;**121**(4):822-828

[6] de Oliveira GC, Solari HP, Ciola FB, Lima ALH, Campos MS. Corneal infiltrates after excimer laser photorefractive keratectomy and LASIK. Journal of Refractive Surgery Thorofare NJ 1995. 2006;**22**(2):159-165

[7] Gelender H, Carter HL, Bowman B, Beebe WE, Walters GR. Mycobacterium keratitis after laser in situ keratomileusis. Journal of Refractive Surgery Thorofare NJ 1995. 2000;**16**(2):191-195

[8] Solomon R, Donnenfeld ED, Holland EJ, Yoo SH, Daya S, Güell JL, et al. Microbial keratitis trends following refractive surgery: Results of the ASCRS infectious keratitis survey and comparisons with prior ASCRS surveys of infectious keratitis following keratorefractive procedures. Journal of Cataract and Refractive Surgery. 2011;**37**(7):1343-1350

[9] Llovet F, de Rojas V, Interlandi E, Martín C, Cobo-Soriano R, Ortega-Usobiaga J, et al. Infectious keratitis in 204 586 LASIK procedures. Ophthalmology. 2010;**117**(2):232-238

[10] Moshirfar M, Welling JD, Feiz V, Holz H, Clinch TE. Infectious and noninfectious keratitis after laser in situ keratomileusis occurrence, management, and visual outcomes. Journal of Cataract and Refractive Surgery. 2007;**33**(3):474-483

[11] Garg P, Chaurasia S, Vaddavalli PK, Muralidhar R, Mittal V, Gopinathan U. Microbial keratitis after LASIK. Journal of Refractive Surgery Thorofare NJ 1995. 2010;**26**(3):209-216

[12] Mittal V, Jain R, Mittal R, Sangwan VS. Post-laser in situ keratomileusis interface fungal keratitis. Cornea. 2014;**33**(10):1022-1030

[13] Karp CL, Tuli SS, Yoo SH, Vroman DT, Alfonso EC, Huang AH, et al. Infectious keratitis after LASIK. Ophthalmology. 2003;**110**(3):503-510

[14] Afsharpaiman S, Zare M, Yasemi M, Jamialahmadi T, Sahebkar A. The prevalence of infectious keratitis after keratorefractive surgery: A systematic review and meta-analysis study. Journal of Ophthalmology. 2020;**2020**:6329321

[15] Schallhorn JM, Schallhorn SC, Hettinger K, Hannan S. Infectious

keratitis after laser vision correction: Incidence and risk factors. Journal of Cataract and Refractive Surgery. 2017;**43**(4):473-479

[16] Feizi S, Jadidi K, Naderi M, Shahverdi S. Corneal interface contamination during laser in situ keratomileusis. Journal of Cataract and Refractive Surgery. 2007;**33**(10):1734-1737

[17] Ortega-Usobiaga J, Martin-Reyes C, Llovet-Osuna F, Damas-Mateache B, Baviera-Sabater J. Interface fluid syndrome in routine cataract surgery 10 years after laser in situ keratomileusis. Cornea. 2012;**31**(6):706-707

[18] Soleimani M, Masoumi A, Farrokhpour H, Keykhaei M, Zeidabadinejad H, Tabatabaei SA. Increased rate of infectious keratitis after PRK in the COVID-19 era: The possible role of face masks. Journal of Refractive Surgery Thorofare NJ 1995. 2022;**38**(2):78-81

[19] Liu J, Guo X, Wei Z, Zhang Y, Zhang Z, Xu X, et al. Infectious keratitis after keratorefractive surgery: Update and review of the literature. Eye & Contact Lens. 2023;**49**(7):275-282

[20] Lazaro C, Perea J, Arias A. Surgical-glove-related diffuse lamellar keratitis after laser in situ keratomileusis: Long-term outcomes. Journal of Cataract and Refractive Surgery. 2006;**32**(10):1702-1709

[21] Liu HY, Chu HS, Chen WL, Hu FR, Wang IJ. Bilateral non-tuberculous mycobacterial keratitis after small incision lenticule extraction. Journal of Refractive Surgery Thorofare NJ 1995. 2018;**34**(9):633-636

[22] Chang MA, Jain S, Azar DT. Infections following laser in situ keratomileusis: An integration of the published literature. Survey of Ophthalmology. 2004;**49**(3):269-280

[23] Semoun O, Bourcier T, Dupas B, Puech M, Maftouhi AE, Borderie V, et al. Early bacterial keratitis after presbyopic LASIK. Cornea. 2008;**27**(1):114-116

[24] de la Cruz J, Behlau I, Pineda R. Atypical mycobacteria keratitis after laser in situ keratomileusis unresponsive to fourth-generation fluoroquinolone therapy. Journal of Cataract and Refractive Surgery. 2007;**33**(7):1318-1321

[25] Vieira AC, Pereira T, de Freitas D. Late-onset infections after LASIK. Journal of Refractive Surgery Thorofare NJ 1995. 2008;**24**(4):411-413

[26] Lu N-J, Qian K, Sorcha ND. Acanthamoeba keratitis after corneal refractive surgery: A case series and literature review. Journal of Refractory Surgical Case Report. 2022;**2**(2):e32-e37

[27] Balasubramanya R, Garg P, Sharma S, Vemuganti GK. Acanthamoeba keratitis after LASIK. Journal of Refractive Surgery Thorofare NJ 1995. 2006;**22**(6):616-617

[28] Lindbohm N, Moilanen JAO, Vesaluoma MH, Tervo TMT. Acinetobacter and *Staphylococcus aureus* ulcerative keratitis after laser in situ keratomileusis treated with antibiotics and phototherapeutic keratectomy. Journal of Refractive Surgery Thorofare NJ 1995. 2005;**21**(4):404-406

[29] Symes RJ, Catt CJ, Males JJ. Diffuse lamellar keratitis associated with gonococcal keratoconjunctivitis 3 years after laser in situ keratomileusis. Journal of Cataract and Refractive Surgery. 2007;**33**(2):323-325

[30] Donnenfeld ED, Kim T, Holland EJ, Azar DT, Palmon FR, Rubenstein JB,

et al. ASCRS White Paper: Management of infectious keratitis following laser in situ keratomileusis. Journal of Cataract and Refractive Surgery. 2005;**31**(10):2008-2011

[31] Tourtas T, Kopsachilis N, Meiller R, Kruse FE, Cursiefen C. Pressure-induced interlamellar stromal keratitis after laser in situ keratomileusis. Cornea. 2011;**30**(8):920-923

[32] Lee V, Sulewski ME, Zaidi A, Nichols CW, Bunya VY. Elevated intraocular pressure-induced interlamellar stromal keratitis occurring 9 years after laser in situ keratomileusis. Cornea. 2012;**31**(1):87-89

[33] Sahay P, Bafna RK, Reddy JC, Vajpayee RB, Sharma N. Complications of laser-assisted in situ keratomileusis. Indian Journal of Ophthalmology. 2021;**69**(7):1658-1669

[34] Kuo CY, Chang YF, Chou YB, Hsu CC, Lin PY, Liu CJL. Delayed onset of pressure-induced interlamellar stromal keratitis in a patient with recurrent uveitis. Medicine (Baltimore). 2017;**96**(48):e8958

[35] Levartovsky S, Rosenwasser G, Goodman D. Bacterial keratitis after [correction of following] laser in situ keratomileusis. Ophthalmology. 2001;**108**(2):321-325

[36] Freitas D, Alvarenga L, Sampaio J, Mannis M, Sato E, Sousa L, et al. An outbreak of *Mycobacterium* chelonae infection after LASIK. Ophthalmology. 2003;**110**(2):276-285

[37] Haq Z, Farooq AV, Huang AJW. Infections after refractive surgery. Current Opinion in Ophthalmology. 2016;**27**(4):367-372

[38] Ortega-Usobiaga J, Llovet-Osuna F, Djodeyre MR, Llovet-Rausell A, Beltran J, Baviera J. Incidence of corneal infections after laser in situ keratomileusis and surface ablation when moxifloxacin and tobramycin are used as postoperative treatment. Journal of Cataract and Refractive Surgery. 2015;**41**(6):1210-1216

Chapter 3

Alternative Treatment Approaches in Bacterial Keratitis

Lional Raj Daniel Raj Ponniah

Abstract

Microbial keratitis can cause unilateral blindness, which can occur after ocular trauma and subsequent infection, causing unilateral blindness in 1.5 to 2 million corneal ulceration cases globally per year, particularly in developing and tropical countries. The conventional treatment options are largely topical in a loading dose regimen. This chapter enumerates the recent advances in its management. Parenteral, and intracorneal, intrastromal antimicrobial injections are attempted as adjuvants in refractory cases. Novel drug reservoir contact lenses have higher bioavailability by creating an antimicrobial lake with increased tear film exchange through the fenestration. Sustained release intrastromal antimicrobial implants for the treatment of deep corneal infections and abscesses have increased efficacy. An intensive loading dose with topical agents could be reduced with alternative approaches, thus reducing the treatment burden and improving patient compliance.

Keywords: bacterial keratitis, bacterial corneal ulcer, drug-eluting contact lens, microemulsions, photoactivated chromophore for keratitis, intrastromal injection, drug-depository contact lens, corneal cross-linking

1. Introduction

Bacterial keratitis (BK) is an acute condition perverting the vision to cause blindness if untreated acutely. Currently, microbial keratitis may be epidemic and may exceed 2 million cases per year worldwide [1]. In the US among one million infectious keratitis around 58,000 cases of BK were reported [2]. Bacterial infection was predominant in developed countries whereas developing countries face challenges in corneal infections due to fungal, bacterial, and other origins. One of the reports from the south Indian cities claimed 113 MK in 100,000 individuals [3].

Generally, the bacterial keratitis in its acute condition, the treatment was initiated with a time lag due to delayed presentations in developing countries. In addition, Gram staining and culture sensitivity with antibiogram are time-consuming procedures with challenging availability at all primary or secondary eye care setups.

Hence, while initiating the therapy the size of the ulcer or the intensity of the severity would have progressed to another grade. An intensive approach would impact early recovery and prevent the incidence of smaller ulcers becoming larger corneal ulcers.

Surgical modalities of therapeutic Deep Anterior Lamellar Keratoplasty (DALK), and therapeutic penetrating keratoplasty in cases of fulminating bacterial keratitis, impending perforation, or actual perforation are not discussed in this chapter. Other alternate modalities of treatment of BK are given importance and are discussed here.

2. Bacterial keratitis management

2.1 Standard medical treatment

Bacterial keratitis is generally treated instantaneously upon its diagnosis by clinicians. After confirming bacterial etiology, the patient should be started on broad-spectrum antibiotic therapy, covering both gram-positive and negative bacteria. Once the culture results are available after 48 to 72 hours, the treatment may be switched to targeted antibacterial therapy if an empirical therapy is not responsive. To treat peripheral ulcers without visual axis involvement (<3 mm), monotherapy with fourth generations of quinolones is initiated. In the case of larger and deep stromal ulcers, it is better to start two antibacterials to prevent irreversible vision-threatening sequelae [4].

2.1.1 Topical antibiotics

The topical fluoroquinolones are available as 0.3% ciprofloxacin, 0.3% ofloxacin, 0.5% moxifloxacin, and 0.3% gatifloxacin. They are primarily instilled as monotherapy. Recently, growing resistance has been noted for ciprofloxacin and ofloxacin; hence, moxifloxacin and gatifloxacin are being used with more efficacy in managing bacterial keratitis [5].

The most common cephalosporins implicated is bacterial keratitis with topical cefazolin 5% (fortified). It is best suitable for non-penicillinase-producing gram-positive bacteria.

Aminoglycosides including fortified topical tobramycin 0.3% or gentamicin 0.3%, or amikacin 1 g/ml injection are very effective against gram-negative bacteria, streptococci, and staphylococci but have a very limited response against pneumococci. Fortified cefazolin and tobramycin as combination therapy are most commonly employed as an alternative to monotherapy with fourth-generation quinolones in bacterial keratitis. Fortified vancomycin 5% is very active against methicillin-resistant *staphylococcus aureus* (MRSA).

Poor drug availability due to pre-corneal factors and deeper penetration into corneal layers remains a challenge with topical therapy and hence alternative treatment options are needed to be explored.

The role of systemic antibiotics in the management of bacterial keratitis is limited. It was used only in endophthalmitis, scleritis, or non-resolving progressive bacterial ulcers. The drugs implicated are ciprofloxacin 750 mg BD or an aminoglycoside with cephalosporin [6].

2.1.2 Steroids

The main treatment is the topical antibiotic for the management of bacterial keratitis and the clinical benefits are appreciable when corticosteroids were used along with topical antibiotics. The topical steroids in the case of microbial keratitis are controversial. Steroids minimize tissue damage by reducing neovascularization, stromal melting, and scarring [7, 8]. Overall pain control and comfort are obvious in steroids that also improve patient compliance [8]. Conversely, steroid therapy may delay epithelial healing and potentiate bacterial keratitis, leading to stromal thinning and melting.

Four clinical trials, including one randomized, placebo-controlled, double-masked trial known as the Steroid for Corneal Ulcer Trial (SCUT), have compared clinical outcomes in bacterial keratitis treated with antibiotics and steroids vs. antibiotics alone [8, 9].

Earlier trials with topical steroids yielded an ambiguous result; however, it gave insight into the subgroup analysis within SCUT patients with low vision patients conveying an appreciable visual improvement at 3 months when compared with placebo, as did patients with invasive Pseudomonas strains. No significant difference in adverse effects was noted between steroid and placebo arms [9].

3. Alternative treatment approaches in bacterial keratitis novel drug delivery methods

Antibiotic eye drops were the most common first-line treatment option and this requires high drug compliance for the therapeutic outcome. The frequent eye drops administration makes them wearisome and thus poor healing.

Exploiting contact lenses for constant drug delivery (zero-order kinetics) was highly challenging. The soft contact lenses exhibiting the feature of drug uptake and release were explored to extend their use in attaining therapeutic index. The pharmacokinetic profile in contact lens drug release is nonlinear kinetics, as there is an immediate drug release and later it tends to decrease to a sub-therapeutic level in the subsequent hours.

Research has also focused on the controlled release of medications from delivery systems incorporated into a contact lens hydrogel material, including copolymerizing the hydrogel and poly (hydroxyethyl methacrylate) (pHEMA) with other monomers.

Hydrogel prototype lenses are used to release the drug in the form of microemulsions. Only first-order kinetics was achieved by manipulating the surface of the contact lenses with the drug-containing liposomes. The physiochemical environment of the human eye with alkaline pH and physiological temperature were the odd factors that prohibit the sustained release of the drug.

Formerly many non-contact lens techniques were attempted in futile to achieve long-term drug release. Ocusert by Alza Corp., Palo Alto, CA, was specifically designed to be placed in the cul-de-sac and had demonstrated zero-order kinetics and it was not widely used except to treat glaucoma, whereas the collagen shields require surgical removal of corneal epithelium to promote corneal re-epithelialization and thereby antibiotic prophylaxis. This method was also not being used due to its hostile natures such as difficulty in self-insert, requiring topical anesthesia, and replacement of a new collagen shield, every 3 days.

As a result, novel drug delivery methods are needed to increase compliance and therefore the efficacy of treatment.

The challenges in achieving the desired sustained release system in an ophthalmic drug were the bioavailability of the drug, the biocompatibility of the contact lenses, absorption and release of the drug in a zero-order kinetics to achieve an extended-release of the drug, etc. In the early 1960s, hydrogel contact lens were introduced and used as a drug-eluting contact lens and as a bandage contact lens. The hydrogel contact lenses as bandage contact lenses were helpful in cornea protection and corneal re-epithelization with antibiotic drops. Unlikely the extended release of antibiotic eye drops could not be established in the hydrogel contact lenses.

A prototype contact lens for sustained drug delivery by incorporating a thin drug-PLGA [Poly (lactic-co-glycolic acid)] film into a pHEMA hydrogel [Poly (2-hydroxyethyl methacrylate)], and this polymer was used in the making of regular contact lenses also. This warrants a regular adjustment of polymer molecular mass and medication concentration in the drug-PLGA film, to reach the zero-order kinetics. This ocular drug delivery system was prominent to maintain therapeutic concentration for about a month. This prototype contact lens design was used as a platform for ocular drug delivery and therapeutic applications. The contact lenses are used as the antibacterial prototype lenses through antibiotic coating with ciprofloxacin-PLGA 65:35 films (pHEMA).

In this prototype contact lens phenomenon, there was an initial drug release in the first 24 hours, followed by this burst the prototype contact lens maintains zero-order kinetics for more than 4 weeks. For instance, 134 μg of ciprofloxacin per day was released constantly to maintain the zero-order kinetics. The ciprofloxacin (23%) was released from the lenses in a month.

A drug-eluting contact lens with a combination of drugs say, moxifloxacin (MF) and dexamethasone (DM), were experimented with. In this study, a polymeric contact lens using chitosan, glycerol, and polyethylene glycol (PEG) was developed along with MF and DM. Drug-loaded contact lenses were tested with a combination of drugs as well as individually, and all three lenses were compared to treatment with individual drug solutions. Both required therapeutic concentration and corneal drug distribution of MF were significant in drug-loaded contact lenses when compared to topically given drug solutions in rabbits and humans. It also features *in vitro* and *in vivo* antimicrobial activity through mucoadhesion by contact lenses [10].

The moxifloxacin in nanoparticles increased the corneal penetration compared to MF in solution. The improved therapeutic effect was obtained when *in situ* gel formation was combined with nanoparticles that is, nanoparticles can also be used to load antibiotics; moxifloxacin nanoparticles show increased corneal penetration. When the liquid gets into contact with the corneal surface, it forms an *in situ* gel that maintains bioavailability [11, 12].

Another breakthrough in nanoparticle research is molecular imprinting. Antibodies were formed through the conversion of nanoparticles into synthetic antibodies equivalent. These antibodies target the lipopolysaccharides in *P. aeruginosa*, in a keratitis model. Methicillin-resistant *Staphylococcus aureus* (MRSA) was also targeted in a similar approach.

Apart from lenses offering the sustained release of drugs, antimicrobial compounds have been incorporated into the lens itself; AGMNA, a metal–organic framework featuring silver (a natural antimicrobial agent), has been developed both for inclusion into the contact lens structure and as a lens disinfecting agent, with high effectiveness and minimal toxicity [13].

In the above study, the Metal–Organic Framework (MOF) of formula {[Ag6(μ3-HMNA)4(μ3-MNA)2]2 – ·[(Et3NH)+]2·(DMSO)2·(H2O)} (AGMNA), a known efficient antimicrobial compound which contains the anti-metabolite, 2-thionicotinic acid (H2MNA), was incorporated in polymer hydrogels using hydroxyethylmethacrylate (HEMA).

pHEMA@AGMNA-1 has antimicrobial activity against the microbial keratitis etiologies gram-negative *P. aeruginosa* and gram-positive *Staphylococcus epidermidis* and

S. aureus. The following organism is incubated with pHEMA@AGMNA-1 discs with % bacterial viability say *P. aeruginosa*, *S. aureus*, and *S. epidermidis* [13]. Furthermore, pHEMA@AGMNA-1 exhibits low toxicity.

3.1 Microemulsions

Microemulsions are another novel method of ocular drug delivery and have shown a promising result in a combined *in vivo* and *in vitro* study [14]. A tiny droplet with a diameter of 10 to 100 nm is formed by the drug with the surfactant. The lipid-water-lipid sandwich of the cornea makes an effective microemulsions delivery [15]. The outer layer of the cornea is a barrier to hydrophilic substances but is lipid-soluble; thus, microemulsions can effectively deliver a drug to the stroma.

Antibiotics can also be similarly delivered to the eye by liposomes, a capsule made of a phospholipid bilayer. Furthermore, Mishra et al. found that contact lenses equipped with liposomes are capable of providing a stable release of antibiotics over 6 days, which was effective against *S. aureus in vitro*.

3.2 Plasma and phage therapy

Plasma and phage therapy was a novel therapeutic option in BK treatment. Plasma is an ionized gas capable of exhibiting antimicrobial properties *via* its ability to produce reactive oxygen species; it also exhibits wound healing and anti-inflammatory properties [16].

Reitberger et al. studied the argon-based plasma therapy and opined that it shall be successfully exploited in combination with antibiotics [16]. Phage therapy involves using a viral bacteriophage to infect and kill bacteria. There was only one study to support the efficiency of phage therapy against *P. aeruginosa* keratitis in mice [17]. Also, a case study reports the efficacy of phage therapy against MRSA keratitis. The effectiveness of phage therapy against a wide number of different non-ocular bacterial colonies has been confirmed by other studies, but there is a need for further investigation focusing specifically on *S. aureus* keratitis isolates.

3.3 Photoactivated chromophore for keratitis-corneal cross-linking (PACK-CXL)

It works on the mechanism of collagen fiber photopolymerization on the corneal tissue to get stiffened by applying a combination of ultraviolet A radiation and a chromophore (riboflavin). This is a non-invasive procedure performed with topical anesthesia.

The photoactivated chromophore and ultraviolet A light have antibacterial properties and are effective in treating infectious keratitis. The antibacterial mechanism involved here is inhibition of microbial replication, intercalation of the chromophore with microbial nucleic acids, RNA damage, DNA damage, cell wall damage, and oxidation of nucleic acid residues by reactive oxygen species, as well as increased resistance of the stiffened cornea to enzymatic damage from the microorganisms. Other potential advantages of UVA and riboflavin application over antibiotics include eliminating ocular surface toxicity and avoiding adherence issues associated with the need for frequent eye drop administration, among others [18].

PACK-CXL with ultraviolet A and riboflavin was applied on the day of diagnosis. According to the Dresden modified protocol, riboflavin 0.1% solution was administered to the cornea every minute for 15 minutes, followed by exposure to 370-nm UVA light (with a fluence of 3 mW/cm^2) from a distance of 1 cm for 30 minutes. Following this, the eye was given a saline rinse and a contact lens was placed. A post-operative regimen of 0.1% fluorometholone acetate eye drops was instilled for 2 days (4 times a day) and for 1 week (3 times a day). The contact lens was removed one day after placement.

The epithelial healing was monitored as a mark of recovery where the patient will receive antibiogram results based on topical antibiotic eye drops along with artificial tear eye drops. During this period, the patient will also wear UV protection glasses. The patient was observed for the presence or absence of corneal ulcer and a comparison was made for treatment response against different time points.

The significance of ulcer healing was moderate in the early weeks of the treatment i.e., from between Day 1 and Week 1. The healing tends to increase over time Month 3 > Month 1 > Week 1. Complete recovery in all treated eyes was accomplished except for four cases due to emergency surgery.

3.4 Thymosin beta 4: a potential novel adjunct treatment for bacterial keratitis

Topical Thymosin beta 4 (Tβ4) was an amino acid protein and it exerts a pharmacological action of promoting wound healing and reducing corneal inflammation when it is used as an adjunct to ciprofloxacin. The mechanism of action was reducing inflammatory mediators and inflammatory cell infiltration that gives an antibacterial activity and wound healing in the experimental model of *P. aeruginosa*-induced keratitis. Tβ4 as a novel therapeutic method has the potential to treat corneal pathogenesis and other infections including immune-based inflammatory diseases [19].

3.5 Novel drug repository contact lens

Ponniah et al. [20] studied a newer drug-delivery mechanism, called the drug-depository contact lens (DDCL; Hyper-CL (Acofilcon A)), and evaluated the effectiveness of DDCLs for bacterial keratitis.

It was an open-label randomized controlled trial that compares the topical antimicrobial eye drops with and without the application of DDCL in treating bacterial keratitis.

The basic principle was fenestration; that is, the topically administered antibiotic drop would migrate through the fenestration holes and reaches the space between the backside of the therapeutic contact lens and the corneal surface. This increased the contact time of antibiotic eye drop and wound, thus enabling relatively speedy recovery when compared to conventional antibiotic eye drop alone.

They evaluated the effects of DDCL using clinical parameter guidelines recommended by the American Academy of Ophthalmology, *viz.*, corneal infiltration size, ulcer size, anterior chamber reactions, corneal haze, visual acuity, and pain. Topical antibiotic Moxifloxacin (0.5%), a Fourth-generation fluoroquinolone having a wide spectrum of antibacterial activity, was used in the study.

In this study, it was observed that corneal infiltration resolution was on day 5 in the antibiotic-only group and day 3 in the DDCL group. Both the groups had lesions healed completely after 2 weeks; however, improvement in terms of healing and pain score was significant in the DDCL group (**Figures 1** and **2**) [20].

DDCL, a therapeutic soft contact lens that was also a repository contact lens, has facilitated the promotion of healing and pain relief in patients suffering from BK. The extended contact of antibiotics over the corneal surface has impacted faster healing of ulcers without an experience of ocular surface toxicity.

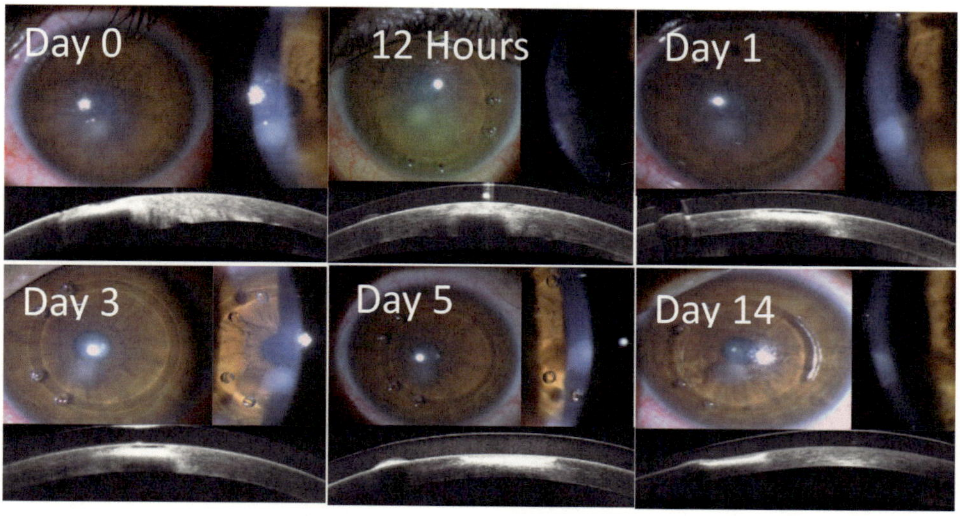

Figure 1.
Corneal ulcer heal in BK infection—DDCL + antibiotics along with corneal OCT.

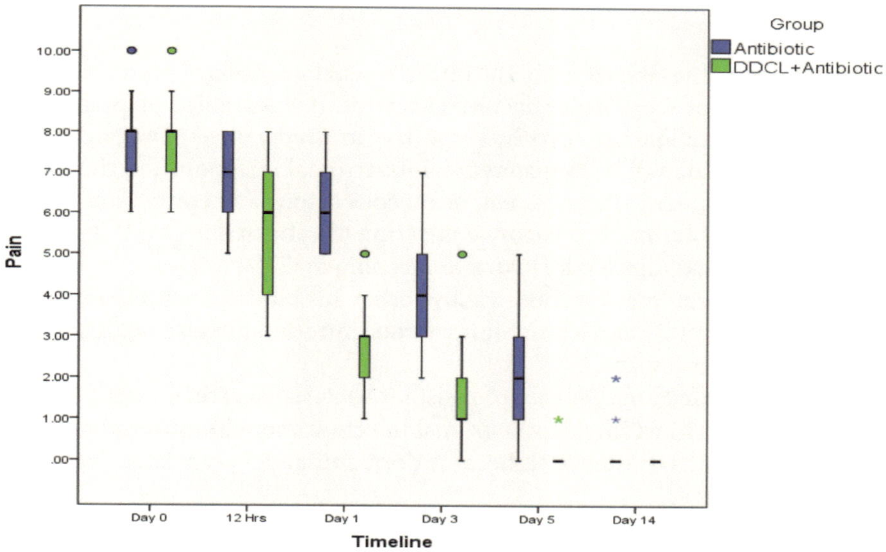

Figure 2.
Changes in pain over time.

3.6 Novel implantable sustained release antibacterial disc

Intra corneal sustained-release dosage forms are novel targeted drug delivery systems to release a drug slowly to maintain a constant drug concentration at the site of action for a specific time with minimum side effects such as ocular surface toxicities.

A novel implantable sustained-release antibacterial disc that provides a likely effect in the treatment of posterior corneal infections and abscesses regarding effective drug penetration and reduced surface toxicities was investigated by the team in South India (**Figure 3**).

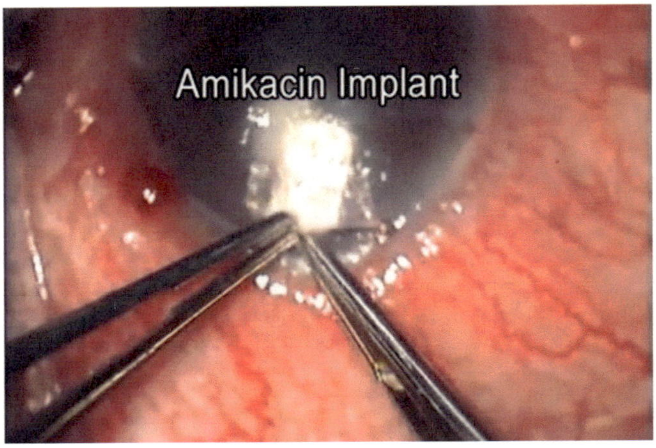

Figure 3.
Implantable sustained release antibacterial disc [21].

3.7 Intrastromal injections with antibiotic agents in the management of bacterial keratitis

Khan et al. were the first to study the intrastromal injections of antibiotic agents in the management of recalcitrant bacterial keratitis. It was studied on patients with infectious crystalline keratopathy secondary to *Streptococcus paranguis*, where cefuroxime 250 μL/mL was administered in intrastromal injection. Yet, the patients initially needed to undergo debridement of mucous plaque and epithelium to expose corneal stroma and biofilm. Intrastromal injection of cefuroxime (1 ml) in the lesion and stroma region was injected by hydration technique [22].

In this case, cefuroxime was chosen above other antibiotics, such as vancomycin, not only for its sensitivity and low inhibitory concentration but also because it is less harmful to the ocular surface.

Liang et al. reported another case of resistant bacterial keratitis. About 0.02 mL of tobramycin (0.3%) in a single intrastromal injection was administered with a 30 G needle. After 6 months, the keratitis became dormant, and 5 years later, there was no sign of a recurrence [23].

Pak et al. was the first to explain triple-bacterial keratitis which was caused by penicillin-resistant *S. aureus*, pan-sensitive *Staphylococcus epidermidis*, and Achromobactin species and its treatment with intrastromal antibiotic injection. When topical treatment failed to treat the keratitis, a new strategy was used and 0.2 mL of 0.5% moxifloxacin was administered intrastromally, precisely at the edge of the infiltrate. The study explained that the complete remission of the keratitis was accomplished with the first dose at the initial and the second dose after 2 weeks [24].

4. Conclusions

Novel approaches are inculcated in the existing bacterial keratitis management to thwart the challenges in disease prognosis rate. Earlier topical antibiotics were the only options for treating bacterial keratitis and surgical management for fulminant keratitis.

The topical antibiotics too have some limitations in terms of bioavailability despite having frequent administration. Novel drug delivery systems were explored to overcome the limitation of topical applications.

These alternative interventions including drug delivery contact lenses, drug repository contact lenses, microemulsions, bacteriophage, pack-CXL, intrastromal injections, etc., provide hope and feasible options for treating bacterial keratitis.

A corneal physician can decide on the various armamentarium tools in addition to intensive topical therapy in treating bacterial keratitis.

Acknowledgements

Thanks go to Dr. Velupillai Ranilakshmi, Prof. Heber Anandan, and Dr. Antonysamy Arulanandham.

Conflict of interest

The authors declare no conflict of interest.

Author details

Lional Raj Daniel Raj Ponniah
Dr. Agarwal's Eye Hospital and Institute of Ophthalmology, Tirunelveli, Tamil Nadu, India

*Address all correspondence to: drlionalraj@gmail.com

References

[1] Ung L, Bispo PJ, Shanbhag SS, Gilmore MS, Chodosh J. The persistent dilemma of microbial keratitis: Global burden, diagnosis, and antimicrobial resistance. Survey of Ophthalmology. 2019;**64**:255-271. DOI: 10.1016/j.survophthal.2018.12.003

[2] Collier SA, Gronostaj MP, MacGurn AK, Cope JR, Awsumb KL, Yoder JS. Beach MJ; Centers for Disease Control and Prevention (CDC). Estimated burden of keratitis–United States, 2010. MMWR. Morbidity and Mortality Weekly Report. 2014;**63**(45):1027-1030

[3] World Health Organization. Guidelines for the Management of Corneal Ulcer at Primary, Secondary and Tertiary Care Health Facilities in the South-East Asia Region. New Delhi: WHO regional office for south-east Asia; 2004 Available from: https://apps.who.int/iris/handle/10665/205174

[4] Wong RL, Gangwani RA, Yu LW, Lai JS. New treatments for bacterial keratitis. Journal of Ophthalmology. 2012;**2012**:831502. DOI: 10.1155/2012/831502

[5] Gokhale NS. Medical management approach to infectious keratitis. Indian Journal of Ophthalmology. 2008;**56**(3):215-220. DOI: 10.4103/0301-4738.40360

[6] Daniell M. Overview: Initial antimicrobial therapy for microbial keratitis. British Journal of Ophthalmology. 2003;**87**(9):1172-1174. DOI: 10.1136/bjo.87.9.1172

[7] Ni N, Srinivasan M, McLeod SD, Acharya NR, Lietman TM, Rose-Nussbaumer J. Use of adjunctive topical corticosteroids in bacterial keratitis. Current Opinion in Ophthalmology. 2016;**27**(4):353-357. DOI: 10.1097/ICU.0000000000000273

[8] Hirano K, Tanaka H, Kato K, Araki-Sasaki K. Topical corticosteroids for infectious keratitis before culture-proven diagnosis. Clinical Ophthalmology. 16 Feb 2021;**15**:609-616. DOI: 10.2147/OPTH.S297202

[9] Srinivasan M, Mascarenhas J, Rajaraman R, Ravindran M, Lalitha P, Glidden DV, et al. Corticosteroids for bacterial keratitis: The steroids for corneal ulcers trial (SCUT). Archives of Ophthalmology. 2012;**130**(2):143-150. DOI: 10.1001/archophthalmol.2011.315 Epub 2011 Oct 10

[10] Gade SK, Nirmal J, Garg P, Venuganti VV. Corneal delivery of moxifloxacin and dexamethasone combination using drug-eluting mucoadhesive contact lens to treat ocular infections. International Journal of Pharmaceutics. 2020;**591**:120023. DOI: 10.1016/j.ijpharm.2020.120023

[11] Lee JW, Somerville T, Kaye SB, Romano V. Staphylococcus aureus keratitis: Incidence, pathophysiology, risk factors and novel strategies for treatment. Journal of Clinical Medicine. 2021;**10**(4):758. DOI: 10.3390/jcm10040758

[12] Upadhyay SU, Chavan SK, Gajjar DU, Upadhyay UM, Patel JK. Nanoparticles laden In situ gel for sustained drug release after topical ocular administration. Journal of Drug Delivery Science and Technology. 2020;**57**:101736. DOI: 10.1016/j.jddst.2020.101736

[13] Rossos AK, Banti CN, Kalampounias AG, Papachristodoulou C, Kordatos K, Zoumpoulakis P, et al.

pHEMA@ AGMNA-1: A novel material for the development of antibacterial contact lens. Materials Science and Engineering: C. 2020;**111**:110770. DOI: 10.1016/j.msec.2020.110770

[14] Bhattacharjee A, Das PJ, Adhikari P, Marbaniang D, Pal P, Ray S, et al. Novel drug delivery systems for ocular therapy: With special reference to liposomal ocular delivery. European Journal of Ophthalmology. 2019;**29**(1):113-126. DOI: 10.1177/1120672118769776

[15] Üstündağ-Okur N, Gökçe EH, Bozbıyık Dİ, Eğrilmez S, Ertan G, Özer Ö. Novel nanostructured lipid carrier-based inserts for controlled ocular drug delivery: Evaluation of corneal bioavailability and treatment efficacy in bacterial keratitis. Expert Opinion on Drug Delivery. 2015;**12**(11):1791-1807. DOI: 10.1517/17425247.2015.1059419

[16] Reitberger HH, Czugala M, Chow C, Mohr A, Burkovski A, Gruenert AK, et al. Argon cold plasma–a novel tool to treat therapy-resistant corneal infections. American Journal of Ophthalmology. 2018;**190**:150-163. DOI: 10.1016/j.ajo.2018.03.025

[17] Fukuda K, Ishida W, Uchiyama J, Rashel M, Kato SI, Morita T, et al. Pseudomonas aeruginosa keratitis in mice: Effects of topical bacteriophage KPP12 administration. PLoS One. 2012;7(10):e47742. DOI: 10.1371/journal.pone.0047742

[18] Gulias-Cañizo R, Benatti A, De Wit-Carter G, Hernández-Quintela E, Sánchez-Huerta V. Photoactivated chromophore for keratitis-corneal collagen cross-linking (PACK-CXL) improves outcomes of treatment-resistant infectious keratitis. Clinical Ophthalmology. 21 Dec 2020;**14**:4451-4457. DOI: 10.2147/OPTH.S284306

[19] Sosne G, Berger EA. Thymosin beta 4: A potential novel adjunct treatment for bacterial keratitis. International Immunopharmacology. 2023;**118**:109953. DOI: 10.1016/j.intimp.2023.109953

[20] Ponniah LR, Ranilakshmi V, Anandan H, Caroline J, Arulanandham A. Novel drug-repository contact lens for prolonging the antimicrobial-cornea interaction for bacterial keratitis treatment: Randomised controlled trial results. BMJ Open Ophthalmology. 2022;**7**(1):e001093. DOI: 10.1136/bmjophth-2022-001093

[21] War on Posterior Corneal Infections, a video presented in 4th Annual Global Video Contest. 2018. Available from: https://www.aao.org/education/clinical-video/war-on-posterior-corneal-infections-2 [Assessed: 7 July 2023]

[22] Khan IJ, Samer H, Saaeha R. Infectious crystalline keratopathy treated with intrastromal antibiotics. Cornea. 2010;**29**(10):1186-1188. DOI: 10.1097/ICO.0b013e3181d403d4

[23] Liang SY-W, Lee GA. Intrastromal injection of antibiotic agent in the management of recalcitrant bacterial keratitis. Journal of Cataract & Refractive Surgery. 2011;**37**(5):960-962, ISSN 0886-3350. DOI: 10.1016/j.jcrs.2011.03.005

[24] Pak CM, Savage DE, Plotnik R, Wozniak RA. Intrastromal antibiotic injection in polymicrobial keratitis: Case report and literature review. Case Reports in Ophthalmology. 2022;**13**(2):550-555. DOI: 10.1159/000525156

Section 2

Non-Infectious Keratitis

Chapter 4

Peripheral Ulcerative Keratitis Associated with Autoimmune Diseases

Marta Świerczyńska, Agnieszka Tronina and Ewa Mrukwa-Kominek

Abstract

Peripheral ulcerative keratitis (PUK) is a destructive inflammatory disease of the juxtalimbal cornea associated with crescent-shaped corneal stromal thinning, epithelial defect, and inflammatory corneal infiltrate. Inflammation of other adjacent tissues, particularly the sclera, is seen quite frequently. Predilection of the peripheral cornea for PUK is explained by its anatomical and physiological characteristics. Both cell-mediated and humoral immunity, in conjunction with the corneal tissue-destroying action of metalloproteinases (MMPs), are implicated in the pathogenesis of PUK. Nearly half of all cases of noninfectious PUK are associated with connective tissue diseases (rheumatoid arthritis (RA) is the most frequent underlying disease) and vasculitis (mostly granulomatous with polyangiitis (GPA)). It is important to determine the etiology and exclude conditions that could mimic PUK e.g., marginal keratitis or Terrien's marginal degeneration (TMD). Therapy should comprise the attenuation of ophthalmic inflammation, but the underlying disease should be treated as a priority. For autoimmune diseases, it is crucial to work closely with internist/rheumatologist to determine an effective immunomodulatory therapeutic approach. PUK is also known to be a potentially devastating and vision-threatening condition that may lead to corneal melting and perforation, requiring surgical intervention. This chapter provides a comprehensive update of current knowledge and therapeutic methods.

Keywords: peripheral ulcerative keratitis, PUK, autoimmune disease, collagen disease, vasculitis, rheumatoid arthritis, granulomatosis with polyangiitis, immunomodulatory therapy

1. Introduction

Peripheral ulcerative keratitis (PUK) is a destructive inflammatory disease, defined as a clinical triad of a rapidly progressive, crescent-shaped area of peripheral corneal thinning, an epithelial defect, and an inflammatory corneal infiltrate. The inflammation often extends to adjacent tissues: conjunctiva, iris, episclera, and sclera [1]. Over time, progressive ulceration can lead to corneal perforation, which in the case of underlying autoimmune etiology has serious ocular morbidity [2]. Although the pathogenesis of

PUK is still not fully understood, it is assumed that peculiar anatomical and physiological features of the peripheral cornea, environmental factors, and cell-mediated and auto-antibody-mediated responses are involved [1, 3–6]. The postulated mechanisms causing PUK are autoimmune reactions to the corneal antigens, circulating immune complex depositions as well as hypersensitivity reaction to exogenous antigens [3].

PUK, after anterior uveitis, is the second most common ocular complication of autoimmune diseases [7]. However, its incidence varies by only 0.2–3 people per million annually [8, 9]. The prevalence is assumed to be higher in the female gender [9], although some studies indicate equal incidence in both sexes [10]. PUK may be caused by a variety of pathological processes, including both ocular and systemic infectious and noninfectious conditions. It is reported that approximately 50% of PUK cases are associated with collagen diseases and various types of vasculitis [11]. PUK can appear at any stage of an already diagnosed underlying systemic disorder and might suggest its exacerbation; however, it may also be the first symptom of a systemic condition. PUK-associated ocular complications and systemic morbidity and mortality can be decreased with timely diagnosis and prompt treatment [4–6].

2. Etiology

PUK may occur because of a variety of ocular and systemic disorders, including infectious and noninfectious conditions. Understanding the following causes of PUK is important for physicians, as PUK can be a rare manifestation of a common disease as well as a common manifestation of a rare disorder. Nearly half of all noninfectious PUK cases are associated with connective tissue diseases, most commonly rheumatoid arthritis (RA). RA is associated with 34% of noninfectious PUK cases; in 50%, it occurs bilaterally and appears in the later stages of the disease [11]. When associated with vasculitis, such as granulomatosis with polyangiitis (GPA), PUK is more often observed as the first manifestation of the underlying condition [12]. Studies suggest that infections are the second most common cause of PUK (about 20% of all cases); therefore, it is essential to rule out probable infectious etiology before starting any immunomodulatory therapy [13].

2.1 Local causes

a. Infectious

- Bacterial (*Staphylococcus*, *Streptococcus*, *Gonococcus*, *Moraxella*, *Hemophilus*, and *Pseudomonas aeruginosa*)
- Viral (Herpes simplex, Herpes zoster, and Epstein-Barr virus)
- Parasite (*Chlamydia trachomatis*)
- Amebic (Acanthamoeba)
- Fungal (*Aspergillus*, *Fusarium*, and dematiaceous fungi)

b. Autoimmune (Mooren's ulcer, allograft rejection, and autoimmune hepatitis)

c. Neurological (neuroparalytic, metaherpetic, and xerophthalmia)

d. Eyelid abnormalities (ectropion, entropion, eyelid tumors, trichiasis, and lagophthalmos)

e. Traumatic (corneal penetrating injury, chemical injury, thermal burns, and radiation injuries)

f. Postoperative (post-LASIK, trabeculectomy, and corneal crosslinking).

2.2 Systemic causes

a. Infectious

- Bacterial (tuberculosis, syphilis, Lyme disease, salmonella gastroenteritis, bacillary dysentery, gonococcal arthritis, and cat scratch disease)

- Viral (Varicella-zoster virus, viral hepatitis, and acquired immune deficiency syndrome)

- Parasite

- Parinaud's oculoglandular fever

b. Autoimmune (**Table 1**)

c. Dermatological diseases (acne rosacea, cicatricial pemphigoid, Stevens-Johnson syndrome, pyoderma gangrenosum, and psoriasis)

d. Malignancies (acute and chronic myelogenous leukemia)

e. Other (hemolytic uremic syndrome, gout, and iatrogenic drugs) [3–6].

	Demographic features	**Systemic findings suggesting the diagnosis**	**Suggestive diagnostic evaluations**
Rheumatoid arthritis (RA)	30–50 years; 3× more common in women	Symmetric pain and swelling in the joints of the hands and feet (rarely large joints), morning stiffness, rheumatoid subcutaneous nodules, myocardial and valvular lesions, rheumatoid nodules in lungs, pulmonary fibrosis, pleuritis, polyneuropathy, carpal tunnel syndrome, vasculitis	RF, anti-CCP; X-ray of joints
Systemic lupus erythematosus (SLE)	16–55 years; 6–10× more common in women	Fever, alopecia without scarring, oral ulcers, butterfly-shaped rash on the face involving the cheeks and bridge of the nose, skin lesions that appear or worsen with the sun exposure, synovitis, pressure pain, morning stiffness	ANA, anti-dsDNA, anti-SM

	Demographic features	Systemic findings suggesting the diagnosis	Suggestive diagnostic evaluations
Sjogren's syndrome	40–60 years; 90% are women	Dry eye and mouth, dryness and itching of the skin, Raynaud's phenomenon	Anti-La, anti-Ro; Schirmer test, TBUT, OSDI
Small—sized vessel vasculitis			
Granulomatosis with polyangiitis (GPA)	45–65 years; more common in men	Epistaxis, ulcerations, sensation of nasal congestion, damage or perforation of the nasal septum, inflammation of the cartilages of the ear or nose, saddle nose, hearing loss, involvement of bronchi, lungs and kidneys	c-ANCA; X-ray or CT of sinuses, lungs; kidney, lung, skin or muscle biopsy
Microscopic polyangiitis (MPA)	50–60 years; slightly higher incidence in men	Fever, weight loss, palpable purpura, livedo reticularis; involvement of lungs and kidneys	p-ANCA, MPO-ANCA; X-ray or CT of chest; kidney, lung or skin biopsy
Eosinophilic granulomatosis with polyangiitis	35–50 years; slightly higher incidence in woman	Asthma, nasal polyps, peripheral neuropathy, transient pulmonary infiltration	MPO-ANCA; eosinophilia; renal function tests; X-ray or CT of sinuses; lung biopsy
Medium-sized vessel vasculitis			
Polyarteritis nodosa	40–60 years; more common in men	Fever, weight loss, palpable purpura, livedo reticularis, skin ulceration, subcutaneous nodules, neuropathy, renal involvement, intestinal ischemia, testicular pain	CTA, MRA, arteriography to confirm microaneurysm; sural nerve or skin biopsy
Large-sized vessel vasculitis			
Giant cell arteritis	70–80 years; 2× more common in women	Acute headache, bilateral temporal scalp hypersensitivity, soreness and swelling in the course of the temporal artery, jaw claudication	ESR and CRP; Doppler ultrasound, CTA, MR to confirm arteritis; temporal artery biopsy
Takayasu's disease	under 50 years; 2–10× more common in men	claudication of the exterminities, absent or asymmetric pulse in the upper extremities, vascular murmurs over constricted arteries, various symptoms depending on the location of the arterial stenosis	USG, CTA, MRA indicating stenosis or obstruction of the aorta, its branches or proximal sections of the limb arteries
Other immune disease			
Behçet's disease, sarcoidosis, inflammatory bowel disease, progressive systemic sclerosis, relapsing polychondritis			

ANA—antinuclear antibody; anti-CCP—anti-cyclic citrullinated peptide; anti-dsDNA—anti-double stranded DNA; anti-SM—anti-Smith; c-ANCA—anti-neutrophil cytoplasmic antibodies; MPO-ANCA—myeloperoxidase anti-neutrophil cytoplasmic antibody; OSDI—ocular surface disease index; p-ANCA—anti-neutrophil cytoplasmic antibodies; RF—rheumatoid factor; TBUT—tear breakup time.

Table 1.
The characteristics of autoimmune causes of PUK [4, 6, 14–16].

3. Pathogenesis of PUK

3.1 Features of the peripheral cornea

The peripheral cornea has unique anatomical and physiological features, some of which make it more susceptible to hypersensitivity reaction, autoimmune processes, and ulcerations [1]. Different from the central part of the cornea, the peripheral cornea has a greater thickness (up to 0.7 mm), and the epithelium is firmly adherent to the underlying basement membrane [17]. Epithelial stem cells are more concentrated, have the highest proliferation rate whereas endothelial cells have maximum myogenic activity [17, 18]. Moreover, higher levels of the cell surface-associated glycoprotein Mucin-4 (MUC-4) gene, which has epithelial-protective activity and is responsible for regulating the renewal and differentiation of epithelial cells, have been found in the corneal periphery [19]. Furthermore, it has less innervation, and therefore sensitivity is lower in this region [18].

Differently from the avascular central cornea, where the main nutritional sources are the tear film and aqueous humor, the limbus and peripheral cornea obtain nutrients from the vascular arcade that originates from the anterior ciliary arteries extending approximately 0.5 mm into the clear cornea [20]. Perilimbal vascular and lymphatic arcades, along with the adjacent conjunctiva, provide a reservoir of different inflammatory cells and cytokines [1, 3].

As a result of tight collagen bundle packing and vascular architecture at the periphery of the cornea, there is an accumulation of high molecular weight compounds (such as IgM, complement component 1 (C1)) and immune complexes, which are unable to diffuse into the central cornea from the limbal vessels [21, 22]. Besides, compared to the central cornea, there is a higher density of Langerhans' cells, which are highly potent antigen-presenting dendritic cells [22].

3.2 B-cell and antibodies

Patients with RA demonstrate loss of normal B-cell tolerance for their own antigens; some have serum IgM directed against their own IgG (RF), and the immune complexes aggregate at the corneal periphery causing complement activation and corneal damage [1]. Anti-CCP antibodies, present in some RA patients, are associated with a more severe presentation of PUK [23]. In SLA, impaired immune tolerance triggers the production of ANA that form immunocomplexes by which the clearance of apoptotic cells is impaired and subsequently causes profound tissue damage [24].

In GPA, ANCA also binds to both monocyte and neutrophil receptors, increasing the release of destructive enzymes and proinflammatory cytokines [25] (in the course of various corneal inflammatory diseases, including PUK, upregulated expression of interleukin (IL)-6, IL-1b and tumor necrosis factor (TNF)-α is important) [3]. Among patients with PUK during RA and GPA, antibodies targeting directly the corneal epithelium have been identified [26, 27].

Besides the production of antibodies, B-cells are involved in producing cytokines that affect pathological T-cell response, regulate Th1/Th2 balance, and participate in presenting antigenic peptides via major histocompatibility complex (MHC) class II molecules [28].

3.3 Complement and innate immunity

Circulating antigen-antibody complexes act on C1, the first element of the classical complement activation pathway [29]. The large size of C1 inhibits its diffusion through the cornea, so it persists at the periphery and corneal stroma [21]. During the activation of complement cascade, C3a and C5a polypeptides are formed, demonstrating chemotactic activity, particularly on neutrophils and eosinophils. Ultimately, the complement system causes stromal destruction and lysis of cell membranes [30, 31]. Studies of corneas affected by PUK have shown a large number of various proinflammatory cells of the innate immune system, e.g., neutrophils, mast cells, plasma cells, eosinophils, which are a source of destructive and collagenolytic enzymes that trigger corneal damage [3].

3.4 T-cell immunity

T-cell response is crucial in protection against pathogens but also plays an important role in immunopathological conditions, e.g., the number of CD4 cells is significantly greater among patients with RA [32]. Adaptive T-cell-mediated immunity has been shown to be involved in PUK formation. T-cells can cause tissue damage either directly or through dysregulated autoantibody and proinflammatory cytokine production [3].

3.5 Matrix metalloproteinases

Metalloproteinases (MMPs) are proteolytic enzymes that cause disruption and disintegration of specific extracellular matrix components. MMPs can be divided according to substrate specificity: collagenases, gelatinases, stromelysins, matrilysins, membrane-type MMPs, and others. The release of cytokines such as IL-1 from inflammatory cells enables stromal keratocytes to produce MMP-1 and MMP-2. The imbalance between MMPs and their respective tissue inhibitors (TIMPs) results in high collagenase activity, increased tissue destruction, ulceration as well as disruption of the tissue repair process by breaking down the newly formed noncrosslinked collagen [33].

MMP-1 (produced by macrophages and fibroblasts) and MMP-8 (produced by neutrophils and invading inflammatory cells near the limbus) play a pathogenic role in the course of PUK, initiating the hydrolysis of fibrillar type 1 collagen, the main component of corneal stroma. The gelatinases (MMP-2, -9) can cleave basement membrane components (collagen type IV, VII; fibronectin, laminin) and stromal collagen types IV, V, VI, the core protein decorin, and denatured collagens [34].

4. Clinical presentation

The majority of PUK occurs unilaterally and affects one segment of the cornea, while it rarely presents in both eyes, in such cases, the lesions are usually asymmetrical [13]. The eye redness, photophobia, tearing, and pain are the initial symptoms of PUK. Pain is an important feature and can vary in intensity. Deterioration of visual acuity can occur in the active phase of the disease as a result of inflammation or in the chronic phase secondary to corneal astigmatism with corneal opacity [4].

Slit lamp examination demonstrates peripheral, crescentic destructive inflammation at least 2 mm from the limbus, associated with epithelial defect and corneal thinning. The leading edges are undermined, infiltrated, and de-epithelialized. The involvement of the lower part of the cornea is reported to be prevalent compared to the upper part. The spread is circumferential and occasionally central. The ulceration initially involves the superficial one-third of the cornea and may enlarge over time resulting in corneal perforation. It should be noted that the epithelial defect will predispose to secondary infection [4, 13].

Analysis of anterior segment optical coherence tomography (AS-OCT) is useful in the monitoring of disease activity and the evolution of changes. In the active phase, the absence of corneal epithelium, scrambled appearance of the anterior stroma, and heterogeneous stromal reflectivity are observed. As the inflammation intensity declines, irregular hyporeflective epithelium, a smoother anterior stroma, and a homogeneous hyperreflective stroma can be seen. On the other hand, healed PUK lesion is characterized by a filled corneal defect with a hyporeflective thick epithelium, a demarcation line, and the persistence of the hyperreflective underlying stroma [35, 36].

PUK may clinically present as:

a. Acute, subacute, or chronic peripheral keratitis with ulceration, stromal thinning, and infiltration involving juxtalimbal cornea; hypopyon may be present.

b. Inflammation, in addition to the juxtalimbal cornea, may additionally involve the adjacent conjunctiva, iris, episclera, and sclera, as is particularly often seen when the cause of PUK is autoimmune. Concomitant scleritis (e.g., nodular scleritis, necrotizing scleritis) can exacerbate the course of PUK and increase the risk of complications. In addition, the intensity of keratitis correlates with the course of scleritis, which can be explained by the similar underlying pathological process of collagenolysis in both cases.

c. Healing or healed PUK with a recovered epithelial defect and peripheral corneal thinning. The cornea exhibits diffuse corneal neovascularization and scarring, which can significantly impair visual acuity (**Figures 1–4**).

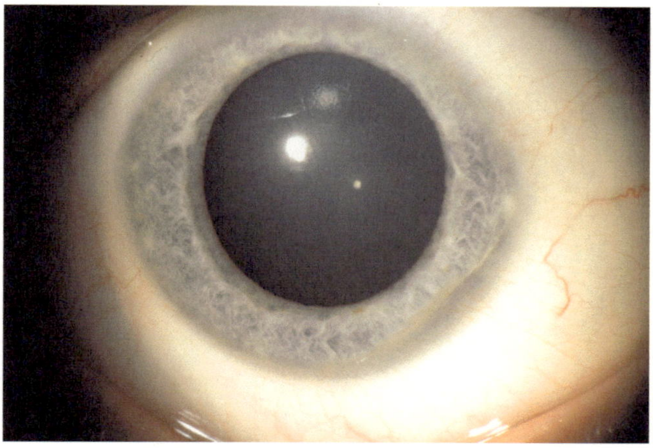

Figure 1.
Crescent-shaped peripheral corneal thinning.

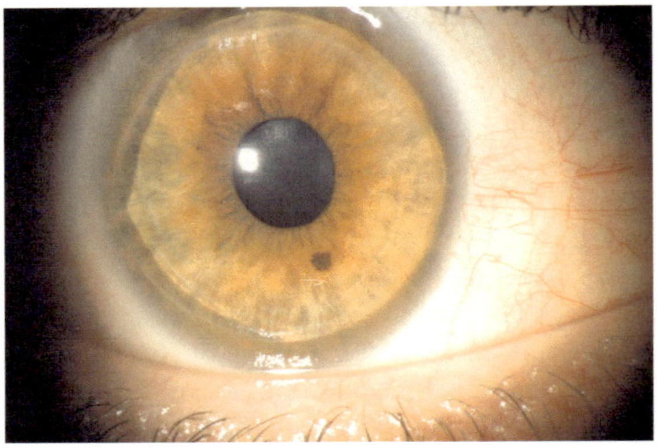

Figure 2.
360 degrees of peripheral corneal thinning.

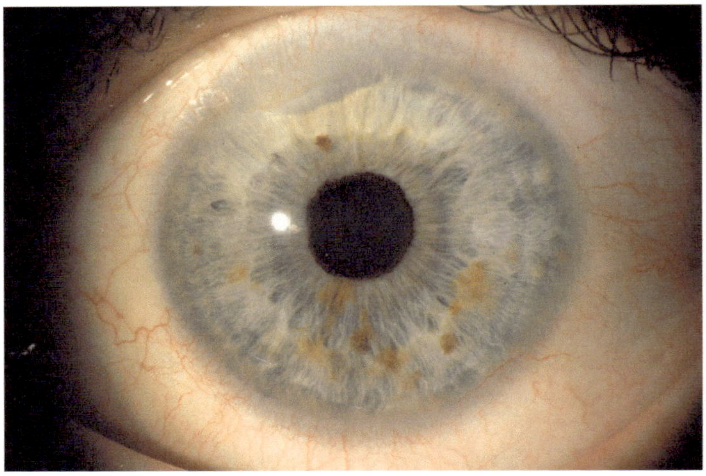

Figure 3.
Sectorial corneal thinning with superficial vascularization.

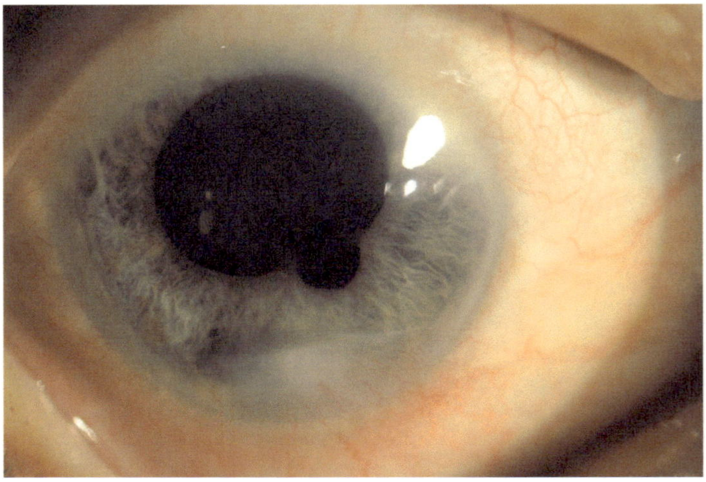

Figure 4.
Peripheral corneal scarring and vascularization. Posterior synechiae due to PUK-associated iritis.

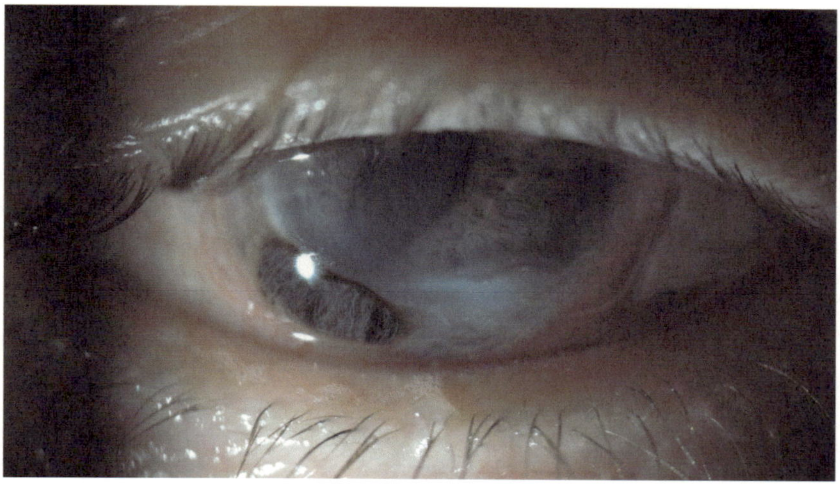

Figure 5.
Corneal perforation and iris tissue prolapse.

d. Corneal perforation or impending perforation is uncommon but is the most serious complication of PUK. Occasionally, accompanying iris prolapse in the area of corneal defect may be observed (**Figure 5**) [5].

5. Differential diagnoses

The differential diagnosis of PUK should include inflammatory conditions (e.g., marginal keratitis and catarrhal infiltrates, phlyctenulosis, rosacea-associated keratitis, MGD-associated keratitis, peripheral infectious keratitis, vernal keratoconjunctivitis). Furthermore, local damage from improperly fitted contact lenses, exposure keratitis, trichiasis, and lid malposition can implicate peripheral corneal diseases [4–6].

a. Marginal keratitis represents an immune response to staphylococcal antigens and can appear either in the course of symptomatic blepharoconjunctivitis or asymptomatic eyelid colonization [37]. Moreover, catarrhal infiltrates emerge secondary to blepharitis and meibomianitis caused by other bacteria (e.g., *Hemophilus*, *Moraxella*, and *Streptococcus*) [38]. Following an immune response to toxins produced by bacteria causes circumscribed infiltrates to deposit at the points of contact of the eyelids to the peripheral cornea [39]. A lucid interval of clear cornea between the infiltrates and the limbus is present, unlike in PUK and phlyctenulosis. Marginal keratitis responds quickly to topical treatment, while PUK, despite receiving topical ophthalmic therapy, may worsen due to other untreated underlying diseases [40].

b. Phlyctenulosis is another immune-mediated peripheral corneal lesion observed primarily in the course of longstanding staphylococcal blepharoconjunctivitis. Phlyctenules are subepithelial nodules that initially appear in the limbus and extend toward the cornea later in the disease. Both marginal keratitis and corneal phlyctenulosis have a similar clinical presentation to PUK and can be difficult to differentiate during ulcerative stages. However, unlike PUK, their symptoms are less severe and usually self-limited [41].

c. Compared to marginal keratitis, herpetic infection begins with an epithelial defect, and then subepithelial infiltrates appear. HSV-induced keratitis may be associated with minor pain due to decreased corneal sensation due to infected corneal neurons [42].

When diagnosing PUK, it is also important to consider noninflammatory corneal disorders associated with peripheral corneal thinning or opacification such as peripheral corneal degeneration, e.g., Terrien's marginal degeneration (TMD), senile furrow degeneration, pellucid marginal degeneration.

a. TMD is distinguished from PUK by the presence of intact epithelium while the juxtalimbal corneal stroma is progressively thinning. TMD usually begins in the upper quadrant of the cornea as fine punctate stromal opacities; superficial neovascularization is present in most cases, and lipid deposits emerge at the ends of vessels over time. A characteristic feature of TMD is a clear gray line of demarcation between the normal cornea and the affected area. The thinned zone can slowly expand circumferentially, causing irregular astigmatism. Patients with this type of degeneration do not report pain [43, 44].

b. Senile furrow degeneration reveals as thinning in the lucid interval between an arcus senilis and limbus, mainly in older individuals. Unlike PUK, the epithelium remains intact, and infiltration and inflammation are absent. Besides, corneal vascularization is absent, which is a distinctive feature of TMD. The furrow is shallow with sloping central and peripheral edges, and the progression of lesions is remarkably slow [4].

MU is a rare, idiopathic form of peripheral corneal ulceration. This can present as unilateral, slowly progressive lesions in older adults and bilateral, rapidly progressing ulcers in younger adults. MU occurs without a specific general underlying disease likely to cause PUK, and it is an exclusion diagnosis. MU is more common in Africa, China, and India; it shows an association with viral exposure (hepatitis C), helminthic infections, HLA-DR17, and DQ2 antigens. The pathological process begins with the involvement of the peripheral cornea, spreads circumferentially, and then centrally with overhanging edges. A distinctive feature of MU, unlike PUK, is the absence of scleritis and the pain being more intense, poorly tolerated, and inadequate in relation to the size of the ulceration [4, 13, 45, 46].

6. Medical management

Prompt treatment of PUK and, in particular, the underlying disease is crucial in order to reduce mortality with ocular and systemic morbidity [11, 40]. The main purposes of PUK treatment are to reduce inflammation, minimize stromal loss, obtain epithelial healing, and prevent infection [4, 40].

6.1 Topical treatment

a. Lubricating eye drops belong to the primary management of PUK. They improve the quality of the tear film, reduce discomfort, and when used regularly, preservative-free drops contribute to the washout of inflammatory mediators involved in the process of keratolysis from the ocular surface. The frequency of instillation depends on the severity of the patient's symptoms. Supplementary administration of lubricant ointment formulations, especially overnight, may improve comfort and enhance epithelialization [4, 5].

b. Topical steroids extensively implemented in the treatment of PUK, suppress the local autoimmune response. According to the severity of inflammation, steroids of varying potency can be used:

   - low (e.g., fluorometholone 0.1%, loteprednol etabonate 0.2%, and 0.5%)
   - moderate (e.g., prednisolone sodium phosphate 0.5%, betamethasone 0.1%, and dexamethasone 0.1%)
   - high (e.g., predinosolone acetate 1%).

c. Subconjunctival or periocular administration of steroids may be beneficial in cases of PUK accompanied by scleritis; however, the risk of scleral perforation occurs. The administration of drops is typically started with q.i.d.; the dosage is modified according to the patient's response and is eventually gradually, slowly reduced. However, these should be used with caution, considering the fact that steroids inhibit collagen production and the wound healing process [7, 47–49]. In RA-related PUK, topical steroids have been shown to increase the chances of corneal perforation by inhibiting fibroblast infiltration [4]. Moreover, their chronic use can lead to a number of side effects such as steroid-induced glaucoma, cataract, or increased susceptibility to ocular infections [5].

d. Topical nonsteroidal anti-inflammatory drugs (NSAIDs) (e.g., ketorolac, diclofenac, bromfenac, nepafenac, and flurbiprofen) are used to reduce the inflammation in PUK. However, they have the potential to induce corneal melts or perforation, especially in elderly patients with additional ocular surface disease [50]. Therefore, low-potency steroids applied b.i.d. or t.i.d. in short courses are preferable to NSAID therapy for patients with RA-related PUK and concomitant dry eye syndrome [5].

e. N-acetylcysteine (NAC) 10–20% concentration, applied b.i.d. or t.i.d.. NAC, by chelating MMP-associated calcium or zinc, irreversibly inhibits MMPs. Moreover, NAC reduces the release of proinflammatory cytokines [51].

f. Topical cyclosporine A (CsA) 2% and topical tacrolimus 0.03% are calcineurin inhibitors, they inhibit T-cell function as well as signaling [52]. While CsA shows less efficacy in suppressing the innate immune response in PUK, it is still a useful adjuvant therapy. It enhances ulcer healing, and its topical, unlike general, administration is not associated with nephrotoxicity [53, 54].

g. Progestins (e.g., medroxyprogesterone 1%) have anti-inflammatory activity by binding to glucocorticoid receptors. In addition, by inhibiting neutrophil-related collagenases, they can inhibit corneal stroma degradation and facilitate collagen synthesis [55, 56]. However, there is still a lack of studies demonstrating their efficacy in the treatment of PUK.

6.2 Systemic treatment

Management of PUK associated with autoimmune diseases requires close cooperation between an ophthalmologist and an internist/rheumatologist. Systemic therapy should be directed to both reduce ophthalmological as well as the life-threatening complications of underlying systemic disease [4–6]. The choice of treatment depends on multiple factors including etiology, clinical presentation, severity of disease, systemic co-morbidities, preferred route of drug administration, side effects of medications as well as the patient's general condition including the hematological, liver, and kidney profile [5].

6.2.1 Systemic treatment for the management of ocular morbidity

a. Oral doxycycline is administered at a dose of 100 mg b.i.d. Doxycycline irreversibly inhibits the action of MMPs by chelating metal ions that play catalytic and structural roles. What is more, doxycycline prevents the formation of scar tissue by inhibiting the migration of keratocytes and fibroblasts, instead promoting complete wound surface overlay with epithelial basal cells and the formation of stable stratified epithelium [57, 58].

b. Oral ascorbic acid is taken as an additional treatment, 500 mg b.i.d., for peripheral corneal melting. Animal studies have shown its therapeutic effect on corneal epithelial lesions and influence on the formation of minor corneal opacities after the inflammation has healed [59, 60].

c. Oral NSAIDs (e.g., flurbiprofen, indomethacin) are taken to reduce pain and inflammation for severe cases of PUK, especially those associated with scleritis [5].

6.2.2 Systemic treatment for the management of the underlying systemic condition

The current treatment regimen at the active phase includes application of systemic steroids with their rapid therapeutic effect along with immunomodulatory agents, which are often necessary to induce remission of autoimmune disease. This is followed by gradual tapering of steroids and maintaining the immunomodulatory agent to avoid disease recurrence. Foster et al. found that the mean survival rate in patients having PUK and scleritis in the course of RA, GPA, and SLE is 24.7 years if systemic immunomodulatory therapy is administered versus 10.7 years without this treatment [61].

First-line management of RA-associated PUK involves systemic steroids and a cytotoxic agent (e.g., methotrexate (MTX)) [62]. Second-line agents such as azathioprine and cyclophosphamide are used for severe, refractory PUK cases unresponsive to MTX [63]. Immunosuppressive treatment in the acute phase of GPA is usually initiated with systemic corticosteroids along with cyclophosphamide, and if no improvement is observed, treatment may be changed to rituximab [64].

In pediatric patients, MTX is considered a first-line immunosuppressant in the treatment of underlying systemic treatment, but if it is ineffective second-line cyclosporine is considered [65]. In pregnant women, immunomodulatory therapy should be avoided due to its teratogenic effects, and oral steroids should be used with greater caution [5].

a. Systemic steroids

Due to their availability and quick therapeutic effect, are used as first-line therapy in acute inflammatory diseases. Oral prednisone treatment is usually started with a dose of 1 mg/kg/day (maximum 100 mg/day) and then gradually tapered depending on clinical response [1]. For severe PUK, which threatens vision, intravenous pulses of methylprednisolone (1 g/day for 3 days) are used, followed by a switch to orally administered prednisone and a gradual reduction in dose [48]. Still, the side effects of chronic steroid administration should be kept in mind: glucocorticoid effect, electrolyte disturbances, hypertension, and hyperglycemia. Adjuvant use of H2-blockers to prevent steroid-related gastric ulcers is advisable as well as calcium supplementation to prevent bone density reduction [66].

b. Cytotoxic agents

- Antimetabolites

Methotrexate (MTX) administered typically in a dose of 5–25 mg once a week, inhibits dihydrofolate reductase (DHFR) and therefore decreases DNA synthesis. Its action is on rapidly dividing cells including B and T lymphocytes, making it the widely used immunosuppressive drug in the first-line treatment of PUK in RA. It presents less severe drug toxicity than the majority of other immunosuppressants [1, 67, 68].

Azathioprine is administered by 1–2.5 mg/kg/day; a purine synthesis inhibitor, which inhibits DNA synthesis in proliferating cells. It has been reported that among patients with RA-associated PUK unresponsive to steroid therapy, both MTX and azathioprine show high efficacy. Additionally, azathioprine is considered a much safer but less effective drug than cyclophosphamide [67, 69, 70].

Mycophenolate mofetil is administered as 1–1.5 g twice daily; an inosine-5′-monophosphate dehydrogenase inhibitor, thereby inhibiting the purine synthesis pathway required for replication of lymphocytes. It comes as an effective treatment when combined with steroids. The drug seems to be more effective and safer in the treatment of PUK, compared to MTX and azathioprine, especially in cases where the side effects of the former drugs are not well tolerated [71, 72].

- Alkylating agents

Trigger an irreversible DNA crosslinking, leading to apoptosis in rapidly dividing cells such as T lymphocytes. These drugs are reserved for the treatment of immune disorders unresponsive to steroids and antimetabolites. They have demonstrated efficiency in the treatment of chronic PUK [63].

Cyclophosphamide is administered at a dose of up to 2 mg/kg/d; it has shown good efficacy in the treatment of GPA-related PUK. Treatment of patients with RA-related PUK, in the combination with systemic steroid treatment along with local treatment, has also shown promising results.

Considering its high cytotoxicity, during therapy, morphology should be repeated every 2–3 weeks [64, 67, 73, 74].

Chlorambucil [75].

- T-cell inhibitors

  Cyclosporine A (CsA) administered at a dose of 1.25 mg/kg b.i.d., with an increase by 0.5 mg after 8 weeks and subsequently as per response (maximum daily dose 4 mg/kg). It is a calcineurin inhibitor, suppresses transcription of IL-2, affecting T-cell activity and promotes healing of epithelial defects therefore reducing associated pain. It shows success in the management of bilateral progressive PUK that is not responsive to treatment with the standard agents. However, there is limited application of this drug considering its serious side effects including nephrotoxicity, hepatotoxicity, and increased incidence of lymphoma [52, 67, 76, 77].

  Tacrolimus [78].

c. Biological therapy

- Rituximab

  A monoclonal antibody, interacts with the CD-20 receptor found on the surface of B lymphocytes. This is the most widely used agent for maintaining remission in ANCA-associated vasculitis (e.g., GPA and MPA). It shows to be more potent in maintaining remission compared to azathioprine or cyclophosphamide [79–82].

- TNF-α inhibitors

  Etanercept (decoy receptor for TNF-α); infliximab, adalimumab, golimumab (monoclonal anti-TNF-α antibodies) inhibit the activity of TNF-α (a proinflammatory cytokine released by macrophages and other inflammatory cells) along with the production of MMPs. They are used for PUK refractory to treatment with other immunosuppressive therapeutics. Preliminary studies demonstrate similar efficacy of rituximab and TNF-α inhibitors in the management of PUK in the course of various rheumatologic diseases [4, 5, 83]. Infliximab has the potential to cause serious side effects such as myocardial infarction, pulmonary embolism, deep vein thrombosis, infusion related reactions, and reactivation of tuberculosis [84]. Etanercept is less effective than infliximab and can cause secondary scleritis, which limits its applications in autoimmune diseases [85]. Adalimumab shows a more effective, safer profile and better patient compliance among anti-TNF-α agents [86, 87].

- Tocilizumab

  Anti-IL-6 monoclonal antibody. To date, relatively few studies exist on their efficacy in PUK, but these drugs are likely to have better results than TNF-α inhibitors in PUK that are resistant to standard therapy [29].

7. Surgical management

Treatment of the underlying disease and management of the local inflammation is crucial in cases of PUK associated with an autoimmune etiology. Surgical procedures for PUK should be performed only after adequate immunosuppression, therefore reducing the risk of subsequent corneal graft melts or rejection, recurrence, and exacerbation of the inflammatory changes [4, 5]. However, this is often not possible. In the case of the most severe complication of PUK, corneal perforation, urgent surgical intervention is required despite the current immune status. The surgical method is selected based on the extent of corneal thinning or perforation and the severity of the ocular condition.

Indications for surgical management of PUK:

a. Tectonic—to maintain or restore the integrity of the eyeball when there is significant corneal thinning, descemetocele, impending corneal perforation, or it has already appeared.

b. Therapeutic—as an additional treatment, in case the peripheral ulceration extends, e.g., removal of the adjacent conjunctiva can be performed.

c. Optical—for visual rehabilitation due to severe astigmatism that is not improving with glasses or contact lenses or for the case of contact lens intolerance. Procedures aimed to improve visual acuity should be performed only when PUK is adequately controlled to prevent deterioration of the local disease [4, 88].

7.1 Surgical techniques

a. Conjunctival resection considering the limbal conjunctiva is a reservoir of immune cells, proinflammatory cytokines, and proteolytic enzymes including collagenase, removal of the adjacent conjunctiva in an area involving 2–3 clock hours is among the therapeutic options to limit the inflammation. However, due to the regeneration of the conjunctiva and the reactivation of the immune response, this procedure has limited efficacy [89, 90].

b. Tissue adhesives with subsequent application of a bandage contact lens is a simple and widely used method for treating descemetocele and corneal perforations that are less than 2–3 mm. This corneal stroma enhancement can bridge to subsequent surgical interventions.

    - Cyanoacrylate glue (butyl monomers) has optimal tectonic strength and rapid polymerization making it widely used for the closure of corneal perforations under 3 mm in PUK of autoimmune etiology [91]. Additionally, it acts as a barrier preventing the inflow of inflammatory cells from the conjunctiva [92]. This adhesive remains for at least a month on the corneal surface followed by spontaneous displacement typically due to epithelial healing that occurs beneath [91]. However, since it is not biodegradable, it has the potential to produce foreign body sensation, papillary conjunctivitis (hence the need for a bandage lens application), corneal neovascularization, infection, and tissue necrosis. If the glue enters the anterior chamber, it can cause corneal adhesion to the iris, pupillary block, secondary glaucoma, granulomatous reaction, and cataract [93, 94].

- Fibrin glue is a biological and biodegradable adhesive manufactured from fibrinogen and thrombin (fibrin glue is associated with a significant cost) [95]. The incidence of complications after its use is quite low and includes mostly the formation of granulomas or cysts [96]. Unlike cyanoacrylate glue, it does not have tectonic strength, which is why it is usually used in conjunction with amniotic membrane graft (AMG) [88].

c. Amniotic membrane graft (AMG) provides mechanical support and reduces the risk of corneal perforation. AM contains protease inhibitors, induces apoptosis of inflammatory cells, inhibits cytokine expression in the damaged corneal surface, and inhibits stromal lysis [97]. In addition, it boosts epithelialization and provides nerve growth factor, which facilitates corneal surface regeneration [98]. AMG has been shown to significantly reduce pain symptoms and stabilize visual acuity in up to 50% of patients [99]. Multilayer AMG is used for corneal perforations of less than 0.5 mm in the treatment of PUK of autoimmune etiology. It is absorbed relatively faster in eyes with inflammation, but, if necessary, it is possible to perform repeated AMG [100]. For perforations <3 mm good results have been shown with a combination of fibrin glue and AMG, as well as a lamellar keratoplasty (LK) in combination with AMG [101].

d. Patch graft

- Corneal patch graft

  Crescentic or circular corneal patch graft provides a favorable anatomical result in patients with concomitant autoimmune disease. Vascular ingrowth, chronic epithelial defect, rapid suture loosening, and dissolution of the transplanted tissue are all frequent complications [102]. The new alternative is to use as donor tissue the lenticule obtained during small incision refractive lenticule extraction (SMILE) [103].

- Scleral patch graft

  Scleral tissue from cadaveric eyeballs provides tectonic stability and is often used in conjunction with cyanoacrylate glue. It is an easy, inexpensive, and effective surgical solution for perforations that are 3–5 mm in size [104]. However, like corneal patch graft, it is associated with a high risk of graft vascularization and opacification, postoperative irregular astigmatism and is limited by the availability of donor tissue [88].

- Tenon's patch graft (TPG)

  Tenon's patch graft (TPG) is a simple and affordable method used for perforations of 3–5 mm, benefiting from the autologous nature of the graft [105].

e. Lamellar keratoplasty (LK) like penetrating keratoplasty (PK), LK is relatively expensive, requires a highly trained surgeon, depends on donor tissue availability and is associated with long postoperative care [88]. However, the advantages of LK over PK are the smaller risk of rejection and while avoiding the intraocular procedure (if no perforation is present), reduction of potential development of cataract, glaucoma, and endophthalmitis. Besides, the LK, by increasing the thickness of the host cornea, reduces the risk of future perforation [106].

  - Crescentic lamellar keratoplasty is commonly used in cases of significant thinning of the marginal area of the cornea in the case of PUK. It involves the placement of a ring-shaped lamellar graft on the periphery of the cornea and attachment with sutures to the host cornea. The size of the graft depends on the shape and size of the thinning zone. The visual acuity obtained after this procedure is reported to be significantly better compared to total LK. Several modifications of this technique exist [107].

  - Compressive crescentic (C-shaped) lamellar keratoplasty comprises the use of undersized crescentic donor tissue and tight sutures, causing a flattening perpendicular to the circumference and correcting the steepening and high astigmatism that occurs in the course of the disease [4, 108].

  - Lamellar corneoscleroplasty can restore ocular integrity and maintain the angle structures when scleral melting is present as well [109].

  - Superficial anterior lamellar keratoplasty (SALK): Decentrated large-diameter SALK has the potential to be used successfully in PUK [110].

  - Deep anterior lamellar keratoplasty (DALK) preserves the host endothelium and Descemet's membrane. Decetrated DALK has shown favorable results in PUK with corneal melt [5].

f. Penetrating keratoplasty (PK) is the method of choice in cases of significant corneal thinning or perforation. However, removal of the inflamed peripheral portion of the cornea associated with large-size PKs (9–9.5 mm) carries twice the risk of rejection compared to standard-size grafts due to the proximity of limbal vessels [107, 111]. There is a greater risk of secondary glaucoma from trabecular meshwork damage due to the placement of sutures and anterior adhesions [112]. The risk of rejection further increases due to the presence of an active inflammatory process. It is reported that PKs performed for perforations in the course of PUK of autoimmune etiology have higher rejection rate compared to PKs performed for other reasons, for instance, due to impaired tissue healing [113]. It has been shown that the 6-month average survival of grafts performed for PUK is 20–40%, which requires subsequent PK [63, 114]. To decrease the rejection rate, it is suggested to use small-size tectonic grafts from 3 to 5.5. mm, however, these are associated with worse visual outcomes [107]. In severe cases of PUK associated with PK failure, keratoprosthesis might be considered [115].

8. Conclusions

PUK is a destructive inflammatory disease of the juxtalimbal cornea. This may occur in the course of an autoimmune disease that has already been diagnosed or may be its first manifestation, with serious systemic consequences. The underlying pathogenesis is not fully understood but appears to involve both cell-mediated as well as auto-antibody-mediated components, resulting in the breakdown of peripheral corneal tissue. PUK is potentially devastating and vision-threatening condition that may lead to corneal melting and perforation. However, surgical procedures performed in the management of PUK associated with collagen vascular disease or vasculitis involve various complications and a high incidence of failure.

When dealing with PUK of autoimmune etiology, the collaboration of an ophthalmologist and an internist/rheumatologist is crucial. It is important to control inflammation of the involved ocular tissues, but especially systemic inflammation, through prompt and optimal management including systemic corticosteroids and tailored immunomodulatory drugs. A great glimpse into the future of PUK management is provided by evolving biological therapies with promising results.

Conflict of interest

The authors declare no conflict of interest.

Acronyms and abbreviations

AMG	amniotic membrane graft
ANA	antinuclear antibody
anti-CCP	anti-cyclic citrullinated peptide
anti-dsDNA	anti-double stranded DNA
anti-SM	anti-Smith
AS-OCT	anterior segment optical coherence tomography
C1	complement component 1
c-ANCA	anti-neutrophil cytoplasmic antibodies
CsA	cyclosporine A
DALK	deep anterior lamellar keratoplasty
DHFR	dihydrofolate reductase
GPA	granulomatous with polyangiitis
HSV	Herpes simplex virus
IL	interleukin
LK	lamellar keratoplasty
MHC	major histocompatibility complex
MMP	metalloproteinase
MPA	microscopic polyangiitis
MPO-ANCA	myeloperoxidase anti-neutrophil cytoplasmic antibody
MTX	methotrexate
MU	Mooren's ulcer
MUC4	Mucin-4
NAC	N-acetylcysteine

NSAID	nonsteroidal anti-inflammatory drug
OSDI	ocular surface disease index
p-ANCA	anti-neutrophil cytoplasmic antibodies
PK	penetrating keratoplasty
PUK	peripheral ulcerative keratitis
RA	rheumatoid arthritis
RF	rheumatoid factor
SALK	superficial anterior lamellar keratoplasty
SLE	systemic lupus erythematosus
SMILE	small incision refractive lenticule extraction
TBUT	tear breakup time
TIMP	tissue inhibitor of metalloproteinase
TMD	Terrien's marginal degeneration
TNF	tumor necrosis factor
TPG	Tenon's patch graft

Author details

Marta Świerczyńska[1,2]*, Agnieszka Tronina[3,4] and Ewa Mrukwa-Kominek[1,2]

1 Faculty of Medical Sciences in Katowice, Department of Ophthalmology, Medical University of Silesia, Katowice, Poland

2 Department of Ophthalmology, Kornel Gibiński University Clinical Center, Medical University of Silesia, Katowice, Poland

3 Faculty of Medical Sciences in Katowice, Department of Pediatric Ophthalmology, Medical University of Silesia, Katowice, Poland

4 Department of Pediatric Ophthalmology, Kornel Gibiński University Clinical Center, Medical University of Silesia, Katowice, Poland

*Address all correspondence to: m.swierczynska93@gmail.com

References

[1] Messmer EM, Foster CS. Vasculitic peripheral ulcerative keratitis. Survey of Ophthalmology. 1999;**43**:379-396. DOI: 10.1016/s0039-6257(98)00051-4

[2] Ogra S, Sims JL, McGhee CNJ. Ocular complications and mortality in peripheral ulcerative keratitis and necrotising scleritis: The role of systemic immunosuppression. Clinical & Experimental Ophthalmology. 2020;**48**: 434-441. DOI: 10.1111/ceo.13709

[3] Dana MR, Qian Y, Hamrah P. Twenty-five-year panorama of corneal immunology: Emerging concepts in the immunopathogenesis of microbial keratitis, peripheral ulcerative keratitis, and corneal transplant rejection. Cornea. 2000;**19**:625-643. DOI: 10.1097/00003226-200009000-00008

[4] Tandon R, Galor A, Sangwan VS. Peripheral Ulcerative Keratitis. Cham: Springer International Publishing; 2017. DOI: 10.1007/978-3-319-50404-9

[5] Gupta Y, Kishore A, Kumari P. Peripheral ulcerative keratitis. Survey of Ophthalmology. 2021;**66**:977-998. DOI: 10.1016/j.survophthal.2021.02.013

[6] Hassanpour K, ElSheikh H, R, Arabi A. Peripheral ulcerative keratitis: A review. Journal of Ophthalmic & Vision Research. 2022;**17**:252-275. DOI: 10.18502/jovr.v17i2.10797

[7] Cao Y, Zhang W, Wu J. Peripheral ulcerative keratitis associated with autoimmune disease: Pathogenesis and treatment. Journal of Ophthalmology. 2017;**2017**:7298026. DOI: 10.1155/2017/7298026

[8] McKibbin M, Isaacs JD, Morrell AJ. Incidence of corneal melting in association with systemic disease in the Yorkshire Region, 1995-7. The British Journal of Ophthalmology. 1999;**83**: 941-943. DOI: 10.1136/bjo.83.8.941

[9] Timlin HM, Hall HN, Foot B. Corneal perforation from peripheral ulcerative keratopathy in patients with rheumatoid arthritis: Epidemiological findings of the British Ophthalmological Surveillance Unit. The British Journal of Ophthalmology. 2018;**102**:1298-1302. DOI: 10.1136/bjophthalmol-2017-310671

[10] Sainz de la Maza M, Foster CS, Jabbur NS. Ocular characteristics and disease associations in scleritis-associated peripheral keratopathy. Archives of Ophthalmology. 2002;**120**: 15-19. DOI: 10.1001/archopht.120.1.15

[11] Tauber J, Sainz de la Maza M, Hoang-Xuan T. An analysis of therapeutic decision making regarding immunosuppressive chemotherapy for peripheral ulcerative keratitis. Cornea. 1990;**9**:66-73

[12] Gu J, Zhou S, Ding R. Necrotizing scleritis and peripheral ulcerative keratitis associated with Wegener's granulomatosis. Ophthalmology and Therapy. 2013;**2**:99-111. DOI: 10.1007/s40123-013-0016-1

[13] Sharma N, Sinha G, Shekhar H. Demographic profile, clinical features and outcome of peripheral ulcerative keratitis: A prospective study. The British Journal of Ophthalmology. 2015;**99**:1503-1508. DOI: 10.1136/bjophthalmol-2014-306008

[14] Lin YJ, Anzaghe M, Schülke S. Update on the pathomechanism, diagnosis, and treatment options for rheumatoid arthritis. Cell. 2020;**9**:880. DOI: 10.3390/cells9040880

[15] Fava A, Petri M. Systemic lupus erythematosus: Diagnosis and clinical management. Journal of Autoimmunity. 2019;**96**:1-13. DOI: 10.1016/j.jaut.2018.11.001

[16] Geetha D, Jefferson JA. ANCA-associated vasculitis: Core curriculum 2020. American Journal of Kidney Diseases. 2020;**75**:124-137. DOI: 10.1053/j.ajkd.2019.04.031

[17] Müller LJ, Pels E, Schurmans LR. A new three-dimensional model of the organization of proteoglycans and collagen fibrils in the human corneal stroma. Experimental Eye Research. 2004;**78**:493-501. DOI: 10.1016/s0014-4835(03)00206-9

[18] Müller LJ, Vrensen GF, Pels L. Architecture of human corneal nerves. Investigative Ophthalmology & Visual Science. 1997;**38**:985-994

[19] Gipson IK, Hori Y, Argüeso P. Character of ocular surface mucins and their alteration in dry eye disease. The Ocular Surface. 2004;**2**:131-148. DOI: 10.1016/s1542-0124(12)70149-0

[20] Watson PG. Vascular changes in peripheral corneal destructive disease. Eye (London, England). 1990;**4**:65-73. DOI: 10.1038/eye.1990.7

[21] Mondino BJ. Experimental aspects and models of peripheral corneal disease. International Ophthalmology Clinics. 1986;**26**:5-14. DOI: 10.1097/00004397-198602640-00002

[22] Mondino BJ. Inflammatory diseases of the peripheral cornea. Ophthalmology. 1988;**95**:463-472. DOI: 10.1016/s0161-6420(88)33164-7

[23] Morgan-Warren PJ, Dulku S, Ravindran J. Peripheral ulcerative keratitis as the presenting feature of systemic rheumatoid vasculitis without joint involvement. International Ophthalmology. 2014;**34**:933-935. DOI: 10.1007/s10792-013-9879-3

[24] Squatrito D, Emmi G, Silvestri E. Pathogenesis and potential therapeutic targets in systemic lupus erythematosus: From bench to bedside. Autoimmunity Highlights. 2014;**5**:33-45. DOI: 10.1007/s13317-014-0058-y

[25] Shiuey Y, Foster CS. Peripheral ulcerative keratitis and collagen vascular disease. International Ophthalmology Clinics. 1998;**38**:21-32. DOI: 10.1097/00004397-199803810-00004

[26] John SL, Morgan K, Tullo AB. Corneal autoimmunity in patients with peripheral ulcerative keratitis (PUK) in association with rheumatoid arthritis and Wegener's granulomatosis. Eye (London, England). 1992;**6**:630-636. DOI: 10.1038/eye.1992.136

[27] Reynolds I, John S, Tullo A. Characterization of two corneal epithelium-derived antigens associated with vasculitis. Investigative Ophthalmology and Vision Sciences. 1998;**39**:2594-2601

[28] Nakken B, Munthe LA, Konttinen YT. B-cells and their targeting in rheumatoid arthritis—Current concepts and future perspectives. Autoimmunity Reviews. 2011;**11**:28-34. DOI: 10.1016/j.autrev.2011.06.010

[29] Dominguez-Casas LC, Sánchez-Bilbao L, Calvo-Río V. Biologic therapy in severe and refractory peripheral ulcerative keratitis (PUK). Multicenter study of 34 patients. Seminars in Arthritis and Rheumatism. 2020;**50**:608-615. DOI: 10.1016/j.semarthrit.2020.03.023

[30] Quintana LF, Kronbichler A, Blasco M. ANCA associated vasculitis: The journey to complement-targeted therapies. Molecular Immunology. 2019; **112**:394-398. DOI: 10.1016/j.molimm.2019.06.018

[31] Metzemaekers M, Gouwy M, Proost P. Neutrophil chemoattractant receptors in health and disease: Double-edged swords. Cellular & Molecular Immunology. 2020;**17**:433-450. DOI: 10.1038/s41423-020-0412-0

[32] Rao DA, Gurish MF, Marshall JL. Pathologically expanded peripheral T helper cell subset drives B cells in rheumatoid arthritis. Nature. 2017;**542**:110-114. DOI: 10.1038/nature20810

[33] Visse R, Nagase H. Matrix metalloproteinases and tissue inhibitors of metalloproteinases: Structure, function, and biochemistry. Circulation Research. 2003;**92**:827-839. DOI: 10.1161/01.RES.0000070112.80711.3D

[34] Brejchova K, Liskova P, Cejkova J. Role of matrix metalloproteinases in recurrent corneal melting. Experimental Eye Research. 2010;**90**:583-590. DOI: 10.1016/j.exer.2010.02.002

[35] Bonnet C, Debillon L, Al-Hashimi S. Anterior segment optical coherence tomography imaging in peripheral ulcerative keratitis, a corneal structural description. BMC Ophthalmology. 2020; **20**:205. DOI: 10.1186/s12886-020-01466-1

[36] Garg A, De Rojas J, Mathews P. Using anterior segment optical coherence tomography to monitor disease progression in peripheral ulcerative keratitis. Case Reports in Ophthalmological Medicine. 2018;**2018**: 1-4. DOI: 10.1155/2018/3705753

[37] Mannis M, Holland E. Cornea. 5th ed. Amsterdam: Elsevier Health Sciences; 2021

[38] Taylor PB, Tabbara KF. Peripheral corneal infections. International Ophthalmology Clinics. 1986;**26**:29-48. DOI: 10.1097/00004397-198602640-00004

[39] Ficker L, Seal D, Wright P. Staphylococcal infection and the limbus: Study of the cell-mediated immune response. Eye (London, England). 1989; **3**:190-193. DOI: 10.1038/eye.1989.27

[40] Yagci A. Update on peripheral ulcerative keratitis. Clinical Ophthalmology. 2012;**6**:747-754. DOI: 10.2147/OPTH.S24947

[41] Chung G. Phlyctenular keratoconjunctivitis and marginal staphylococcal keratitis. In: Krachmer JH, Mannis MJ, Holland EJ, editors. Cornea: Fundamentals, Diagnostic, Management. 3rd ed. New York: Elsevier; 2011

[42] Mondino BJ, Brown SI, Mondzelewski JP. Peripheral corneal ulcers with herpes zoster ophthalmicus. American Journal of Ophthalmology. 1978;**86**:611-614. DOI: 10.1016/0002-9394(78)90176-9

[43] Ding Y, Murri MS, Birdsong OC. Terrien marginal degeneration. Survey of Ophthalmology. 2019;**64**:162-174. DOI: 10.1016/j.survophthal.2018.09.004

[44] Keenan JD, Mandel MR, Margolis TP. Peripheral ulcerative keratitis associated with vasculitis manifesting asymmetrically as fuchs superficial marginal keratitis and terrien marginal degeneration. Cornea. 2011;**30**: 825-827. DOI: 10.1097/ICO.0b013e3182000c94

[45] Zelefsky JR, Srinivasan M, Kundu A. Hookworm infestation as a risk factor for Mooren's ulcer in South India. Ophthalmology. 2007;**114**:450-453. DOI: 10.1016/j.ophtha.2006.08.014

[46] Srinivasan M, Zegans ME, Zelefsky JR. Clinical characteristics of Mooren's ulcer in South India. The British Journal of Ophthalmology. 2007; **91**:570-575. DOI: 10.1136/bjo.2006.105452

[47] Araki-Sasaki K, Katsuta O, Mano H. The effects of oral and topical corticosteroid in rabbit corneas. BMC Ophthalmology. 2016;**16**:160. DOI: 10.1186/s12886-016-0339-5

[48] Galor A, Thorne JE. Scleritis and peripheral ulcerative keratitis. Rheumatic Diseases Clinics of North America. 2007;**33**:835-854. DOI: 10.1016/j.rdc.2007.08.002

[49] Virasch VV, Brasington RD, Lubniewski AJ. Corneal disease in rheumatoid arthritis. In: Krachmer JH, Mannis MJ, Holland EJ, editors. Cornea: Fundamentals, Diagnostic, Management. 3rd ed. New York: Elsevier; 2011

[50] Brunton LL, Hilal-Dandan R, Knollmann BC. Goodman and Gilman's the Pharmacological Basis of Therapeutics. 13th ed. New York: McGraw Hill; 2023

[51] Ramaesh T, Ramaesh K, Riley SC. Effects of N-acetylcysteine on matrix metalloproteinase-9 secretion and cell migration of human corneal epithelial cells. Eye (London, England). 2012;**26**: 1138-1144. DOI: 10.1038/eye.2012.135

[52] Kaçmaz RO, Kempen JH, Newcomb C. Cyclosporine for ocular inflammatory diseases. Ophthalmology. 2010;**117**:576-584. DOI: 10.1016/j.ophtha.2009.08.010

[53] Tandon R, Chawla B, Verma K. Outcome of treatment of mooren ulcer with topical cyclosporine a 2%. Cornea. 2008;**27**:859-861. DOI: 10.1097/ICO.0b013e3181702d0c

[54] Zierhut M, Thiel HJ, Weidle EG. Topical treatment of severe corneal ulcers with cyclosporin A. Graefe's Archive for Clinical and Experimental Ophthalmology. 1989;**227**:30-35. DOI: 10.1007/BF02169821

[55] Khan L, Batavia E. Medroxyprogesterone to treat corneal thinning postcurvularia keratitis. Oman Journal of Ophthalmology. 2019;**12**: 194-196. DOI: 10.4103/ojo.OJO_228_2018

[56] Hicks CR, Crawford GJ. Melting after keratoprosthesis implantation: The effects of medroxyprogesterone. Cornea. 2003;**22**:497-500. DOI: 10.1097/00003226-200308000-00001

[57] Smith VA, Cook SD. Doxycycline—A role in ocular surface repair. The British Journal of Ophthalmology. 2004; **88**:619-625. DOI: 10.1136/bjo.2003.025551

[58] Ralph RA. Tetracyclines and the treatment of corneal stromal ulceration: A review. Cornea. 2000;**19**:274-277. DOI: 10.1097/00003226-200005000-00003

[59] Chen J, Lan J, Liu D. Ascorbic acid promotes the Stemness of corneal epithelial stem/progenitor cells and accelerates epithelial wound healing in the cornea. Stem Cells Translational Medicine. 2017;**6**:1356-1365. DOI: 10.1002/sctm.16-0441

[60] Cho YW, Yoo WS, Kim SJ. Efficacy of systemic vitamin C supplementation in reducing corneal opacity resulting from infectious keratitis. Medicine

(Baltimore). 2014;**93**:e125. DOI: 10.1097/MD.0000000000000125

[61] Foster CS, Forstot SL, Wilson LA. Mortality rate in rheumatoid arthritis patients developing necrotizing scleritis or peripheral ulcerative keratitis. Effects of systemic immunosuppression. Ophthalmology. 1984;**91**:1253-1263. DOI: 10.1016/s0161-6420(84)34160-4

[62] Watanabe R, Ishii T, Yoshida M. Ulcerative keratitis in patients with rheumatoid arthritis in the modern biologic era: A series of eight cases and literature review. International Journal of Rheumatic Diseases. 2017;**20**:225-230. DOI: 10.1111/1756-185X.12688

[63] Messmer EM, Foster CS. Destructive corneal and scleral disease associated with rheumatoid arthritis. Medical and surgical management. Cornea. 1995;**14**: 408-417. DOI: 10.1097/00003226-199507000-00010

[64] Ebrahimiadib N, Modjtahedi BS, Roohipoor R. Successful treatment strategies in granulomatosis with polyangiitis-associated peripheral ulcerative keratitis. Cornea. 2016;**35**: 1459-1465. DOI: 10.1097/ICO.0000000000000919

[65] Malik AR, Pavesio C. The use of low dose methotrexate in children with chronic anterior and intermediate uveitis. The British Journal of Ophthalmology. 2005;**89**:806-808. DOI: 10.1136/bjo.2004.054239

[66] Buchman AL. Side effects of corticosteroid therapy. Journal of Clinical Gastroenterology. 2001;**33**: 289-294. DOI: 10.1097/00004836-200110000-00006

[67] Jabs DA, Rosenbaum JT, Foster CS. Guidelines for the use of immunosuppressive drugs in patients with ocular inflammatory disorders: Recommendations of an expert panel. American Journal of Ophthalmology. 2000;**130**:492-513. DOI: 10.1016/s0002-9394(00)00659-0

[68] Gangaputra S, Newcomb CW, Liesegang TL. Methotrexate for ocular inflammatory diseases. Ophthalmology. 2009;**116**:2188-98.e1. DOI: 10.1016/j.ophtha.2009.04.020

[69] Yy DT, Clements PJ, Peter JB. Lymphocyte characteristics in rheumatic patients and the effect of azathioprine therapy. Arthritis and Rheumatism. 1974;**17**:37-45. DOI: 10.1002/art.1780170107

[70] Pasadhika S, Kempen JH, Newcomb CW. Azathioprine for ocular inflammatory diseases. American Journal of Ophthalmology. 2009;**148**:500-509.e2. DOI: 10.1016/j.ajo.2009.05.008

[71] Thorne JE, Jabs DA, Qazi FA. Mycophenolate mofetil therapy for inflammatory eye disease. Ophthalmology. 2005;**112**:1472-1477. DOI: 10.1016/j.ophtha.2005.02.020

[72] Siconolfi L. Mycophenolate mofetil (CellCept): Immunosuppression on the cutting edge. AACN Clinical Issues. 1996;7:390-402. DOI: 10.1097/00044067-199608000-00007

[73] Clewes AR, Dawson JK, Kaye S. Peripheral ulcerative keratitis in rheumatoid arthritis: Successful use of intravenous cyclophosphamide and comparison of clinical and serological characteristics. Annals of the Rheumatic Diseases. 2005;**64**:961-962. DOI: 10.1136/ard.2004.023283

[74] Pujari SS, Kempen JH, Newcomb CW. Cyclophosphamide for ocular inflammatory diseases.

Ophthalmology. 2010;**117**:356-365. DOI: 10.1016/j.ophtha.2009.06.060

[75] Goldstein DA, Fontanilla FA, Kaul S. Long-term follow-up of patients treated with short-term high-dose chlorambucil for sight-threatening ocular inflammation. Ophthalmology. 2002; **109**:370-377. DOI: 10.1016/s0161-6420 (01)00942-3

[76] McCarthy JM, Dubord PJ, Chalmers A. Cyclosporine A for the treatment of necrotizing scleritis and corneal melting in patients with rheumatoid arthritis. The Journal of Rheumatology. 1992;**19**:1358-1361

[77] Lallemand F, Schmitt M, Bourges JL. Cyclosporine A delivery to the eye: A comprehensive review of academic and industrial efforts. European Journal of Pharmaceutics and Biopharmaceutics. 2017;**117**:14-28. DOI: 10.1016/j. ejpb.2017.03.006

[78] Rodrigues-Diez R, González-Guerrero C, Ocaña-Salceda C. Calcineurin inhibitors cyclosporine A and tacrolimus induce vascular inflammation and endothelial activation through TLR4 signaling. Scientific Reports. 2016;**6**:27915. DOI: 10.1038/ srep27915

[79] Hardy S, Hashemi K, Catanese M. Necrotising Scleritis and peripheral ulcerative keratitis associated with rheumatoid arthritis treated with rituximab. Klinische Monatsblätter für Augenheilkunde. 2017;**234**:567-570. DOI: 10.1055/ s-0042-121315

[80] Watkins AS, Kempen JH, Choi D. Ocular disease in patients with ANCA-positive vasculitis. Journal of Ocular Biology, Diseases, and Informatics. 2009;**3**:12-19. DOI: 10.1007/s12177-009-9044-4

[81] Guillevin L, Pagnoux C, Karras A. Rituximab versus azathioprine for maintenance in ANCA-associated vasculitis. The New England Journal of Medicine. 2014;**371**:1771-1780. DOI: 10.1056/NEJMoa1404231

[82] Bonnet I, Rousseau A, Duraffour P. Efficacy and safety of rituximab in peripheral ulcerative keratitis associated with rheumatoid arthritis. RMD Open. 2021;7:e001472. DOI: 10.1136/rmdopen-2020-001472

[83] Mpofu S, Fatima F, Moots RJ. Anti-TNF-alpha therapies: They are all the same (aren't they?). Rheumatology (Oxford, England). 2005;**44**:271-273. DOI: 10.1093/rheumatology/keh483

[84] Huerva V, Ascaso FJ, Grzybowski A. Infliximab for peripheral ulcerative keratitis treatment. Medicine (Baltimore). 2014;**93**(26):e176. DOI: 10.1097/MD.0000000000 000176

[85] Gaujoux-Viala C, Giampietro C, Gaujoux T. Scleritis: A paradoxical effect of etanercept? Etanercept-associated inflammatory eye disease. Journal of Rheumatology. 2012;**39**:233-239. DOI: 10.3899/jrheum.110865

[86] Cordero-Coma M, Méndez RS, Blanco AC. Adalimumab for refractory peripheral ulcerative keratitis. Journal of Ophthalmic Inflammation and Infection. 2012;**2**:227-229. DOI: 10.1007/ s12348-012-0080-z

[87] Korsten P, Bahlmann D, Patschan SA. Rapid healing of peripheral ulcerative keratitis in rheumatoid arthritis with prednisone, methotrexate and adalimumab combination therapy. Rheumatology (Oxford, England). 2017; **56**:1094. DOI: 10.1093/rheumatology/ kex007

[88] Sabhapandit S, Murthy SI, Sharma N. Surgical management of peripheral ulcerative keratitis: Update on surgical techniques and their outcome. Clinical Ophthalmology. 2022;**16**: 3547-3557. DOI: 10.2147/OPTH. S385782

[89] Brown SI. Mooren's ulcer. Treatment by conjunctival excision. The British Journal of Ophthalmology. 1975;**59**: 675-682. DOI: 10.1136/bjo.59.11.675

[90] O-oC E, Jawaheer L, Ramaesh K. Conjunctival resection for peripheral ulcerative keratitis (PUK). Investigative Ophthalmology & Visual Science. 2016; **57**:1261

[91] Weiss JL, Williams P, Lindstrom RL. The use of tissue adhesive in corneal perforations. Ophthalmology. 1983;**90**: 610-615. DOI: 10.1016/s0161-6420(83) 34508-5

[92] Fogle JA, Kenyon KR, Foster CS. Tissue adhesive arrests stromal melting in the human cornea. American Journal of Ophthalmology. 1980;**89**: 795-802. DOI: 10.1016/0002-9394(80) 90168-3

[93] Sridhar MS, Mandal AK, Garg P. Pupillary block glaucoma after tissue adhesive application and anterior chamber reformation with air. Cornea. 2000;**19**:250-251. DOI: 10.1097/ 00003226-200003000-00026

[94] Rohrbach JM, Wohlrab TM, Nölle B. Zyanoacrylatverletzungen des Auges [Cyanoacrylate injuries of the eye]. Der Ophthalmologe. 2000;**97**:878-880. DOI: 10.1007/s003470070013

[95] Spotnitz WD, Mintz PD, Avery N. Fibrin glue from stored human plasma. An inexpensive and efficient method for local blood bank preparation. The American Surgeon. 1987;**53**:460-462

[96] Hüseyin Cagatay H, Gökçe G, Mete A. Non-recurrence complications of fibrin glue use in pterygium surgery: Prevention and management. Open Journal of Ophthalmology. 2015;**9**: 159-163. DOI: 10.2174/187436410150 9010159

[97] Dua HS, Azuara-Blanco A. Amniotic membrane transplantation. The British Journal of Ophthalmology. 1999;**83**: 748-752. DOI: 10.1136/bjo.83.6.748

[98] Touhami A, Grueterich M, Tseng SC. The role of NGF signaling in human limbal epithelium expanded by amniotic membrane culture. Investigative Ophthalmology & Visual Science. 2002;**43**:987-994

[99] Ngan ND, Chau HT. Amniotic membrane transplantation for Mooren's ulcer. Clinical & Experimental Ophthalmology. 2011;**39**:386-392. DOI: 10.1111/j.1442-9071.2010. 02479.x

[100] Solomon A, Meller D, Prabhasawat P. Amniotic membrane grafts for nontraumatic corneal perforations, descemetoceles, and deep ulcers. Ophthalmology. 2002;**109**: 694-703. DOI: 10.1016/s0161-6420(01) 01032-6

[101] Hick S, Demers PE, Brunette I. Amniotic membrane transplantation and fibrin glue in the management of corneal ulcers and perforations: A review of 33 cases. Cornea. 2005;**24**:369-377. DOI: 10.1097/01.ico.0000151547. 08113.d1

[102] Krysik K, Dobrowolski D, Lyssek-Boron A. Differences in surgical management of corneal perforations, measured over six years. Journal of Ophthalmology. 2017;**2017**:1582532. DOI: 10.1155/2017/1582532

[103] Jiang Y, Li Y, Liu XW. A novel tectonic keratoplasty with femtosecond laser intrastromal lenticule for corneal ulcer and perforation. Chinese Medical Journal. 2016;**129**:1817-1821. DOI: 10.4103/0366-6999.186639

[104] Sharma A, Mohan K, Sharma R. Scleral patch graft augmented cyanoacrylate tissue adhesive for treatment of moderate-sized noninfectious corneal perforations (3.5-4.5 mm). Cornea. 2013;**32**: 1326-1330. DOI: 10.1097/ICO.0b013e31829cb625

[105] Sharma N, Singhal D, Maharana PK. Tuck-In Tenon patch graft in corneal perforation. Cornea. 2019;**38**:951-954. DOI: 10.1097/ICO.0000000000001955

[106] Bessant DA, Dart JK. Lamellar keratoplasty in the management of inflammatory corneal ulceration and perforation. Eye (London, England). 1994;**8**:22-28. DOI: 10.1038/eye.1994.4

[107] Lohchab M, Prakash G, Arora T. Surgical management of peripheral corneal thinning disorders. Survey of Ophthalmology. 2019;**64**:67-78. DOI: 10.1016/j.survophthal.2018.06.002

[108] Cheng CL, Theng JT, Tan DT. Compressive C-shaped lamellar keratoplasty: A surgical alternative for the management of severe astigmatism from peripheral corneal degeneration. Ophthalmology. 2005;**112**: 425-430. DOI: 10.1016/j.ophtha.2004.10.033

[109] Burk RO, Joussen AM. Corneoscleroplasty with maintenance of the angle in two cases of extensive corneoscleral disease. Eye (London, England). 2000;**14**:196-200. DOI: 10.1038/eye.2000.53

[110] Artaechevarria Artieda J, Estébanez-Corrales N, Sánchez-Pernaute O. Peripheral ulcerative keratitis in a patient with bilateral scleritis: Medical and surgical management. Case Reports in Ophthalmology. 2020;**11**:500-506. DOI: 10.1159/000508325

[111] Speaker MG, Arentsen JJ, Laibson PR. Long-term survival of large diameter penetrating keratoplasties for keratoconus and pellucid marginal degeneration. Acta Ophthalmologica. Supplement. 1985;**1989**(192):17-19. DOI: 10.1111/j.1755-3768.1989.tb07089.x

[112] Wu S, Xu J. Incidence and risk factors for post-penetrating keratoplasty glaucoma: A systematic review and meta-analysis. PLoS One. 2017;**12**(4): e0176261. DOI: 10.1371/journal.pone.0176261

[113] Maeno A, Naor J, Lee HM. Three decades of corneal transplantation: Indications and patient characteristics. Cornea. 2000;**19**:7-11. DOI: 10.1097/00003226-200001000-00002

[114] Jhanji V, Young AL, Mehta JS. Management of corneal perforation. Survey of Ophthalmology. 2011;**56**: 522-538. DOI: 10.1016/j.survophthal.2011.06.003

[115] Jerez-Peña M, Salvador-Culla B, de la Paz MF. Bilateral Boston keratoprosthesis type 1 in a case of severe Mooren's ulcer. European Journal of Ophthalmology. 2021;**31**:NP33-NP38. DOI: 10.1177/1120672120909768

Chapter 5

Dry Eye Disease: Chronic Ocular Surface Inflammation

Anna Nowińska

Abstract

Ocular surface inflammation is one of the major features of dry eye disease (DED) according to the definition proposed by the Tear Film and Ocular Surface Society (TFOS) International Dry Eye Workshop (DEWS) in 2007 and 2017. This chapter discusses the potential pathomechanism of the DED vicious cycle and focuses on the role of chronic inflammation and flares in DED pathophysiology. Ocular inflammation may be regarded as both a cause and effect of DED. The current understanding of the mechanism responsible is that the repeating desiccating stress accompanied by hyperosmolarity induces the immune system reaction, leading to the chronic inflammation and apoptosis of ocular surface cells. On the cellular level, there is growing evidence from experimental, animal, and human studies that Th17 lymphocytes play a crucial role in DED pathogenesis. Also, potential methods of anti-inflammatory methods of treatment are discussed, such as eye lubricants, autologous serum eye drops, topical steroids, oral and topical immunomodulation drugs, and N-acetylcysteine (NAC). Understanding the role of inflammation on the cellular and molecular level may lead to improve treatment options for patients. A new approach to DED treatment should be focused to target not only symptoms but also break the pathological dry eye cycle.

Keywords: dry eye disease, ocular surface, ocular inflammation, meibomian gland dysfunction, vicious cycle, eye lubricants

1. Introduction

Dry eye disease is a multifactorial disease of the ocular surface characterized by a loss of homeostasis of the tear film and accompanied by ocular symptoms, in which tear film instability and hyperosmolarity, ocular surface inflammation and damage, and neurosensory abnormalities play etiological roles [1].

Historically, dry eye was mostly considered to be caused by a simple tear deficiency. According to the current definition of the disease, proposed by the Tear Film and Ocular Surface Society (TFOS) International Dry Eye Workshop (DEWS) in 2017, inflammation is one of the major features of the disease accompanied by tear film instability and hyperosmolarity, ocular surface damage, and neurosensory abnormalities. The proposed mechanism of the disease is the self-perpetuating vicious cycle, in which the loss of homeostasis of the tear film plays a major role. The mechanism was broadly introduced in 2007, further adopted by the TFOS DEWS II committee, and remains the leading concept of DED pathophysiology

IntechOpen

[2, 3]. Meibomian gland dysfunction (MGD) is at the center of the vicious cycle of DED. As shown in **Figure 1**, MGD is a key trigger of tear film instability, inflammation, ocular surface apoptosis, and neurosensory abnormalities. Understanding the pathophysiology of DED has significant implications for the methods of diagnosis and methods of treatment. Anti-inflammatory therapies are already available in DED treatment, but understanding their role and differences among them is crucial in successful patient management.

2. Epidemiology, forms, severity, symptoms, signs, and risk factors of DED

DED remains one of the global health problems characterized by the significant impact on the quality of life of patients. It has a global prevalence ranging from 20 to 50%. Data on the prevalence of DED reported over the last 10 years vary widely, which is related to, among others, different standardization of study groups, the lack of uniform diagnostic criteria, the selection of subjective tests (questionnaires of vision quality), and ocular surface examinations to confirm the DED diagnosis. The results of studies based on subjective symptoms indicate the prevalence of DED in the range from 5 to 50%, while studies based on ocular tests indicate the prevalence of up to 75% of the population. International epidemiological studies have estimated the prevalence of DED from 5% to 30% in the population over 50 years of age. The disease is more common in women (1.3–1.5 times more prevalent than in men) and Asians, and its prevalence increases with age [4].

There are two major forms of DED: evaporative DED (EDE) and aqueous deficient dry eye (ADDE). EDE is a predominant form of DE responsible for about 70% of cases. MGD is considered to be the main cause of EDE. MGD is at the center of the vicious cycle of DED. International workshop on MGD defines MGD as a chronic

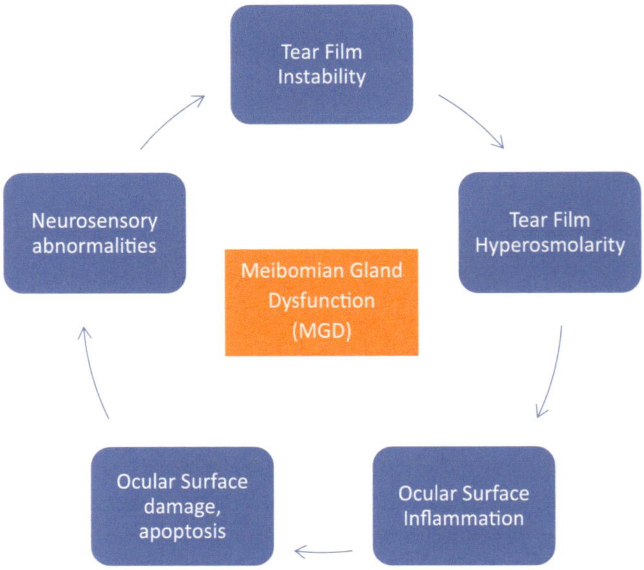

Figure 1.
The simplified vicious cycle of DED based on [1–3].

diffuse abnormality of MG that is commonly characterized by terminal duct obstruction or qualitative or quantitative changes in glandular secretion [5]. Key pathophysiological features of MGD are gland blockade due to hyperkeratinization, ductal stenosis, and chronic stagnation of the meibum. That ultimately leads to gland atrophy and alternations in the lipid tear film layer. MGD may be considered a key trigger of tear film instability, inflammation, apoptosis, and neurosensory abnormalities.

In terms of severity, the predominant forms of DED are mild and moderate. Severe cases are mostly related to systemic, autoimmune diseases (such as rheumatoid arthritis, polyarteritis nodosa, systemic sclerosis), Sjogren syndrome (Sjogren syndrome dry eye; SSDE), and graft-versus-host disease (GVHD).

The impact of DED on the quality of patients' life is significant. This disease has been shown to have a negative impact on patient's daily activities. Due to DED, affected patients may experience decreased productivity as a result of irritating and chronic symptoms. There are several studies underlining the relationship between DED and sleep disorders or depression [6, 7]. Major complaints include pain, eye irritation, foreign body sensation, blurred vision, burning, dryness or watery eyes, fluctuating vision, and photophobia.

If symptoms are accompanied by ocular signs, namely homeostasis markers including decreased tear breakup time (TBUT), increased hyperosmolarity, and positive ocular surface staining the diagnosis of DED may be made. Further, division based on ocular signs includes evaporative and aqueous deficiency DED, as presented in **Figure 2**.

Risk factors of DED were established based on studies with different evidence levels. The epidemiology committee of TFOS DEWS II gathered all risk factors and

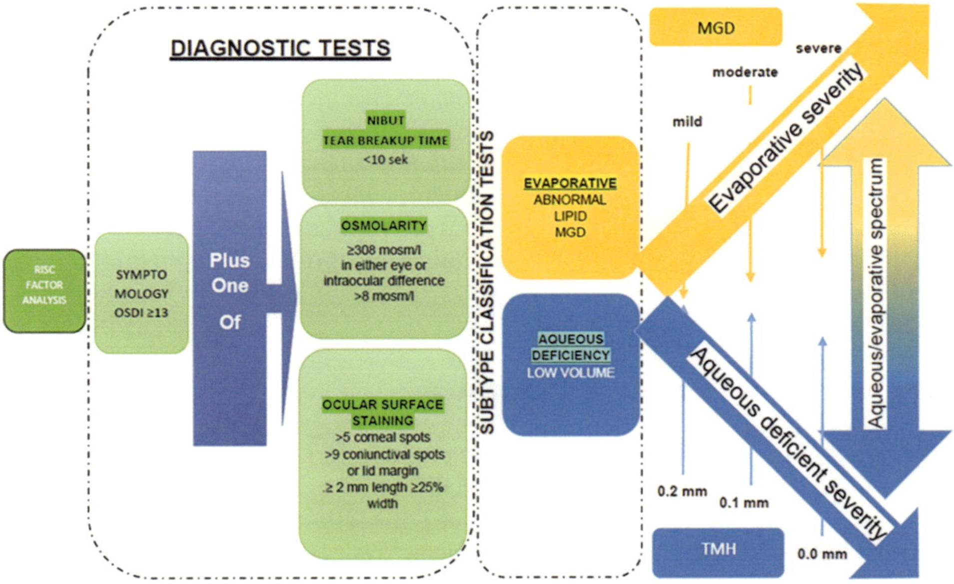

Figure 2.
Diagnostic algorithm of a patient with DED. OSDI—ocular surface disease index; NIBUT—non-invasive tear break up time; MGD—meibomian gland dysfunction; TMH—tear meniscus height; the following sequence of diagnostic tests is recommended: NIBUT, osmolarity test, FBUT with fluorescein (fluorescein tear break up time), ocular surface staining. The diagnostic algorithm is based on the TFOS DEWS II methodology recommendation [8].

Risk factor	Non-modifiable	Modifiable
Consistent	Aging Female sex Asian race Meibomian gland dysfunction Connective tissue diseases Sjögren Syndrome	Androgen deficiency Computer use Contact lens wear Hormone replacement therapy Hematopoietic stem cell transplantation Environment: pollution, low humidity, sick building syndrome Medications: antihistamines, antidepressants, anxiolytics, isotretinoin
Probable	Diabetes Rosacea Viral infection Thyroid disease Psychiatric conditions Pterygium	Low fatty acids intake Refractive surgery Allergic conjunctivitis Medications: anticholinergic, diuretics, beta-blockers
Inconclusive	Hispanic ethnicity Menopause Acne Sarcoidosis	Smoking Alcohol Pregnancy Demodex infestation Botulinum toxin injection Medications: multivitamins, oral contraceptives

Table 1.
DED risk factors established by TFOS DEWS II [4].

divided them into mostly consistent, probable, or inconclusive factors. Factors were also stratified into non-modifiable and modifiable risk factors [4]. The risk factors of DED were presented in **Table 1**.

DED is a disease of many etiological factors, multiple forms, and different severity; therefore, the various management and therapeutic options according to disease form and severity should be considered. Also, regarding the strong association with indoor and outdoor environmental factors, the management and therapy report committee recommends the following strategies, as a part of the initial management of the disease, education regarding the condition, its management, treatment, and prognosis, modification of the local environment, education regarding potential dietary modifications (including oral essential fatty acid supplementation), and identification and potential modification/elimination of offending systemic and topical medications [9].

3. The role of ocular surface inflammation

Understanding the role of inflammation on the cellular and molecular level may lead to improve treatment options for DED patients. Ocular inflammation may be regarded as both a cause and effect of DED. The current understanding of the mechanism responsible is, that the repeating desiccating stress accompanied by hyperosmolarity induces the immune system reaction leading to the chronic inflammation and apoptosis of ocular surface cells. It is important to acknowledge, that different form of DED, such as SS-DED (SS—Sjogren syndrome) and non-SS DED are related to various inflammatory microenvironment. Also, there are significant differences between an acute and chronic state of DED in term of the inflammatory response.

It is also worth emphasizing that regardless of the underlining cause, DED and ocular surface allergy (OA) share common pathognomonic pathways [10]. The chronic and acute reaction of the immune system in atopy, OA, and DED is related to ocular inflammation on the cellular level and its impact on the molecular homeostasis. Inflammatory biomarkers, which are significantly elevated in both conditions include matrix metalloproteinase-9 (MMP-9), Interferon-gamma (INFγ), IL-1α, IL-2, IL-6, IL-8, IL-17, and IL-22. Moreover, cytokines previously regarded as specific to OA are also elevated in DED, and those include IL-4, IL-5, and IL-13. MMP-9 is a proteolytic enzyme, expressed by eosinophils, correlated to the epithelial, and conjunctival cells interruption. MMP-9 level may be assessed in DED and OA patients using commercially available tests. IFN-γ is an inflammatory cytokine secreted by numerous cells such as epithelial cells, CD+T cells, and NK cells. It is one of the major indicators of the ocular surface inflammation. IL-17, IL-22, and IL-6 are the known effector cytokines of Th17 lymphocytes, which are characteristic for both DED and OA [11].

In vivo confocal microscopy (IVCM) allowed us to broaden our knowledge regarding the cellular changes in DED. Specific changes are as follows: the increased stromal nerve thickness and tortuosity, the decreased density of basal epithelial cells, stromal keratocytes, and subbasal nerves, and the presence of dendritic cells, leukocytes, activated keratocytes, and increased level of epithelial and stromal reflectivity [12, 13]. All those features revealed by the IVCM exam, which are characteristic for DED provides a direct, clinical proof, the inflammation plays a crucial role in DED pathogenesis.

On a molecular level, it has been established that proinflammatory cytokines (IL-1α, IL-1β, IL-2, IL-4, IL-5, IL-6, IL-13, IL-17, IL-22, TNFα, tumor necrosis factor α, and INFγ) are over-expressed in the tear film and ocular surface of patients DED [14].

3.1 Cytokines

Inflammation in DED may begin as an acute immune reaction in response to desiccating stress. Mitogen-activated protein (MAP) kinases and NF-κB (nuclear factor kappa-light-chain-enhancer of activated B cells) play a crucial role in initiating and maintaining the immune reaction, leading to the release of pro-inflammatory cytokines, such as TNF-α, IL-1β, and IL-6 on the ocular surface. Activation of toll-like receptor 4 (TLR4) also causes the activation and secretion of pro-inflammatory cytokines, such as IL-1β. At the same time, regardless of the TLR4-mediated pathway, the release of reactive oxygen species (ROS) induces activation of caspase-8 and NLRP3 inflammasome, also promoting the IL-1β release. The process leads to increased expression of MMP-9, a proteolytic enzyme known to break the epithelial corneal barrier and cause punctate keratitis.

3.2 CD+ T cells

There is growing evidence from experimental, animal, and human studies that CD+ T cells play a crucial role in DED pathogenesis. The initiating factor results in the loss of the ocular surface immune homeostasis, and the activation of CD4+ T cells are the leading factors of the tear film instability, hyperosmolarity, ocular surface damage, and neurosensory abnormalities. It is well proved that CD+ T cells differentiate in response to the local microenvironment of cytokines and are defined by their transcription factor expression. With an excess concentration of INFγ and IL-12, CD+ T cells differentiate into Th1 lymphocytes, while in the concentration of Il-6 and TGF-β (transforming growth factor beta), they may differentiate into Th17 lymphocytes. Further, ocular surface damage is caused by proinflammatory cytokines released by Th1 and Th17 lymphocytes, which stimulate the production of MMP-3, and MMP-9. Th17 lymphocytes produce Il-17, which damages the epithelial barrier function and causes apoptosis. Moreover, Th17 lymphocytes are characterized by phenotypic and functional plasticity, which lineage throughout the disease initiation, perpetuation, and sustention. Th17 cells are plastic and can differentiate into Th1 or Th2 subsets depending on environmental stimuli. Recently a new, autoimmune model of DED pathogenesis was proposed based on the concept of Th17 cells mediated disruption of ocular surface immune homeostasis that leads to DED [14]. This model is presented in **Table 2**.

3.3 Differences in inflammatory response in relation DED form and chronicity

There is a difference between an acute and chronic DED in terms of the inflammation activation. Chronic DED is principally mediated by effector memory of Th17 cells because Th17 cells persist in chronic phase of DED. After the resolution of acute inflammation on the ocular surface, a part of effector Th17 cells pool (both eTh17 and eTh17/1 cells) converts into long-lived memory Th17 cells (mTh17). This population of cells is responsible for chronic inflammation. Based on animal studies it was proved, that aged mice (12–14 months) develop a more severe DED than in young mice (6–8 weeks). Aged mice had increased frequencies of conjunctival and draining lymph nodes Th17 cells compared to young mice [15]. Therefore, anti-IL-15 was proposed to reduce the memory of Th17 cells and further the severity of DED.

There is also a difference between immune response in Sjogren (SS-DED) and non-Sjogren DED (non-SS DED). The main feature of SS-DED is the lymphocytic infiltration of the lacrimal glands. The subpopulation of cells consists of primarily CD4+ T cells with minor number of B cells. Several immune mechanisms are common for both DED forms, including Th17 cells activation and overexpression of cytokines such as IL-6, IL-17, and IL-22. However, there is a significant difference in the levels of

1. Hyperosmolar stress, desiccating stress			
2. Induction of adaptive Th17 cells immunity in the ocular surface			
2.1. Release of TNF-α, IL-1β, and IL-6 by mucosal lining cells	2.2. Ocular surface infiltration of monocytes, macrophages, NK cells	2.3. Activation of antigen-presenting cells (APC) on the corneal and conjunctival epithelium	2.4. Lymphatic vessels formation
3. Reaction in the draining lymph nodes			
3.1. T cell priming and Th17 cells differentiation	3.2. Dysfunction of inflammation-limiting regulatory T cells (Treg)	3.3. Expansion and full activation of Th17 cells	3.4. Th 17 cells humoral activation: IL-17, IFN-γ
4. Peripheralization of effector Th17 cells			
5. Ocular surface damage, punctate epitheliopathy caused by Th17 cells through humoral response: IL-17, IFN-γ, and granulocyte-macrophage colony-stimulating factor (GM-CSF)			

Table 2.
The autoimmune model of DED pathogenesis based on [14].

CXCL chemokine (chemokine C-X-C motif) ligand family and macrophage inflammatory proteins chemokine family. Above are highly expressed in SS-DED compared to non-SS DED. Paired box protein Pax-6 (PAX6) is one of the conjunctival protein biomarkers associated with an increased ocular surface damage. Downregulation of PAX6 in SS-DED was significantly related with epithelial damage [11].

3.4 Clinical demonstration of ocular surface inflammation

Resembling other chronic inflammatory conditions, patients with DED have inflammatory flares, typically with rapid exacerbation of symptoms such as redness, eye irritation, and blurred vision. It is postulated that acute inflammation related to DED flare begins with a nonspecific innate immune response, which is usually followed by a slower but more specific adaptive immune response [16]. Various tests are used in scientific studies and clinical practice to assess the level of ocular surface inflammation in patients. Analysis of tear film cytokines and chemokines using ELISA or LUMINEX systems, flow cytometry of conjunctival epithelial cells, impression cytology, or confocal microscopy are rather used in clinical studies. In daily practice, a simplified qualitative test of MMP-9 and lissamine green staining may be used. Lysamine green is a vital dye, which stains epithelial cells only if the cell membrane is damaged, irrespective of the presence of mucin. The result correlates with the level of inflammation on the ocular surface. Examples of ocular surface irritation are presented in **Figure 3**.

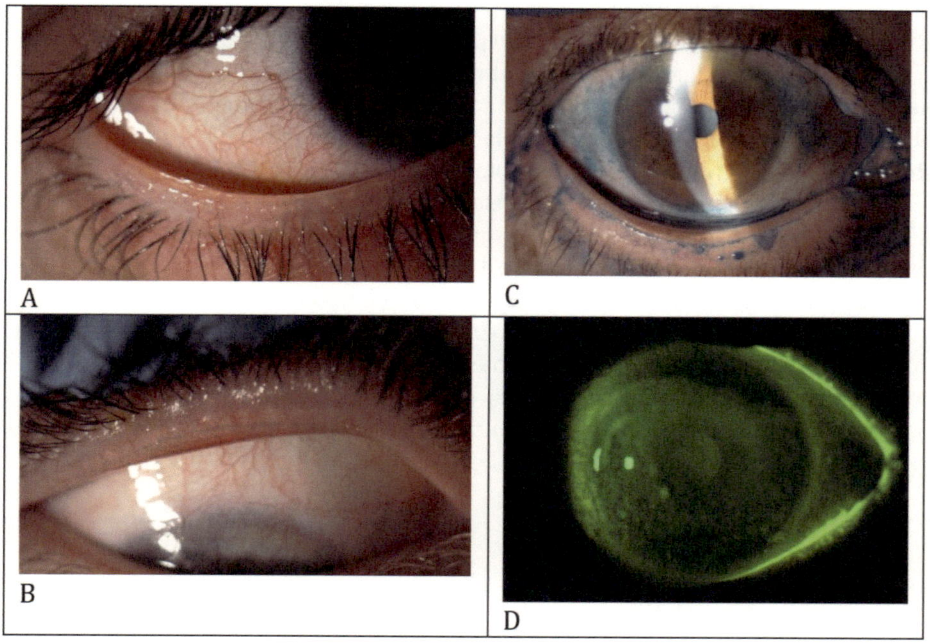

Figure 3.
Ocular surface photos demonstrating inflammation related to DED. a. Slit lamp photo (mag. 10×). Note the visible vascularization of the eyelid margin and conjunctival superficial irritation. b. Slit lamp photo (mag. 10×, installation of lysamine green). Note the plugging of the meibomian glands, vascularization, and Marx line stained with lissamine green. c. Slit lamp photo (mag. 10×, after installation of lysamine green). A positive score of lissamine green staining in a patient with severe dry eye. d. (mag. 10×, after installation of fluorescein; blue-yellow filter applied). A positive score of fluorescein staining showed punctate keratopathy and breaks in the tear film layer.

4. Anti-inflammatory potential of DED treatment methods

4.1 Eye lubricants

Eye lubricants have different properties, which vary between formulas and significantly influence the final effectiveness of treatment. These are viscosity, pH, osmolarity, and electrolyte concentration. Additionally, eye lubricants may contain preservatives, osmotic agents, osmoprotectants, bioprotectants, antioxidants, lipids, amino acids, and inactive agents, such as buffers. Historically, DED was considered to be largely due to tear insufficiency and was treated by prescribing tear replacement products, but these products do not target the underlying pathophysiology of DED. The group includes natural polymers such as HPMC, synthetic polymers (PVP), carbomer gels, and paraffin ointments. To enhance lubrication and prolong the retention time on the ocular surface, a variety of viscosity-enhancing agents are frequently incorporated into such formulas. The main disadvantage of this group of eye drops is the short time of relief of symptoms for the patient, most of them also contain preservatives.

It is already well recognized that chronic exposure of the ocular surface to preservatives induces toxicity and adverse changes to the ocular surface. There are multiple *in vitro* and *in vivo* studies demonstrating that BAK can induce corneal and conjunctival epithelial cell apoptosis, damage the corneal nerves, delay corneal wound healing, induce squamous metaplasia, interfere with tear film stability, and also can cause loss of goblet cells [17–19].

Hyaluronic acid is worth mentioning because its viscosity depends on shear rate and due to its non-Newtonian properties, it mimics the tear film behavior. When open, the eye benefits from a higher tear viscosity to prevent tear film breakup, whereas a lower tear viscosity during blinking prevents damage to the epithelial surface. Moreover, by binding to the CD44 receptor Hyaluronic acid provides enhancement of corneal epithelium healing, improvement of the ocular surface function and protection, and also restoration of the morphology and distribution of goblet cells [20, 21].

The new formulas of eye lubricants usually have complex compositions and treat not only symptoms but are designed to aim at the causes of the disease—hyperosmolarity, inflammation, and ocular surface damage.

The trehalose properties are worth underlining because it is unique in terms of high water retention capabilities but also has the dual properties of both bioprotection and osmoprotection. Trehalose has a protective effect against inflammation in DED. It suppresses proinflammatory cytokines, such as IL-1, 2, 6, 17, TNF-α, as well as proteolytic enzymes (MMP-9), and cell keratinization, which was proved in vitro, in animal, and human studies [22–26].

4.2 N-acetylcysteine (NAC)

NAC is a mucolytic agent but also possesses antioxidant and anti-inflammatory properties. It inhibits cytokine release and suppresses adhesion molecule and nuclear factor kappa-B (NF-κB) expression. The most common concentration in clinical settings in patients with DED and MGD ranges from 5 to 10% topical [27].

4.3 Serum eye drops

In recent years, attention has been paid to autologous peripheral blood serum (PBS), umbilical cord serum (UCS), and platelet-rich plasma (PRP). In clinical settings, autologous serum eye drops are usually applied in concentrations ranging from 20 to 100%. The composition may be regarded to be similar to natural tears, by the content of factors, such as epidermal growth factor (EGF), nerve growth factor (NGF), fibronectin, and vitamins. It has a positive effect on the regeneration of epithelial cells and also has the potential to reduce the activity of inflammatory cytokines and increase the production of mucin and the number of goblet cells [9].

4.4 Topical steroids

Topical corticosteroids are one of the most potent topically applied anti-inflammatory drugs to treat ocular inflammation. Topical corticosteroids are effective in reducing inflammation by stopping the inflammatory cascade at various levels, including (intercellular adhesion molecule 1) ICAM-1-mediated cell adhesion, reducing cytokines, chemokines, MMPs expression, induction of lymphocyte apoptosis, proliferation of fibroblasts, and collagen deposition. Corticosteroids increase the synthesis of lipocortins that block phospholipase A2 and inhibit histamine synthesis in mast cells. The drugs are widely used in all ocular diseases involving inflammation including keratitis, uveitis, ocular allergy, blepharitis, scleritis, and more. One should be aware of the differences among steroids related to the anti-inflammatory potential, drug duration of action, and the potential to incuse adverse events. There are several potential options in ophthalmic setting available such as hydrocortisone 3.35 mg/ml, 0.5% loteprednol etabonate, 0.1% fluorometholone acetate, 0.1% dexamethasone, 0.5% prednisolone acetate, and 0.05% difluprednate. However, soft corticosteroids (such as hydrocortisone 3.35 mg/ml, fluorometholone, or loteprednol 0.5%) may be ideal for the treatment of inflammatory flares in DED and may be considered mainstream anti-inflammatory therapy. Soft steroids have lower to no negative risks of ocular hypertension, cataracts, and infectious diseases, especially when used for a short duration (3–8 weeks).

The use of corticosteroids in DED has been shown to reduce the signs and symptoms associated with DES and prevent DES flares in many non-randomized trials in the clinical setting. Recently, two systemic reviews on the efficacy of topical administration of corticosteroids for the management of DED were published [28, 29]. The main conclusions are a good safety profile of topical steroids and the following benefits: provide small to moderate degrees of symptom relief beyond lubricants, small to moderate degrees of symptom relief beyond cyclosporin A (CsA), and less certain about the effects of steroids on improved tear film quality or quantity. Authors of both systemic reviews underline the need for randomized, controlled trials with larger sample sizes to provide higher-quality evidence to establish the role of steroids in DED.

Topical corticosteroid of limited duration is recommended in DED treatment as a "step 2" option recommended by the TFOS DEWS II guidelines [9].

4.5 Non-glucocorticoid immunomodulators (0.05–0.2% cyclosporin CsA, lifitegrast 5%, azithromycin, 0.03% tacrolimus)

Cyclosporine is a fungal antimetabolite that inhibits IL-2 activation of lymphocytes. Lifitegrast is a small molecule integrin antagonist, which acts as a competitive antagonist to block binding between lymphocyte function-associated antigen 1 (LFA-1) and ICAM-1. Azithromycin and tacrolimus are macrolide antibiotics that have immunosuppressive activity.

All immunomodulators have been proven to provide some degree of positive impact in experimental, animal, and human studies in DED, which solely proves the role of inflammation in DED. The exact treatment dosage and duration are not fully established and this matter requires more randomized clinical trials, as underlined by the TFOS DEWS II committee [9].

4.6 Oral diet supplementation

Essential fatty acids (EFAs) are believed to modulate systemic inflammation; however, the exact impact on inflammation is complex and not fully understood. At present oral EFAs, supplementation is recommended by the guidelines and is believed to support the anti-inflammatory effect of DED [9].

4.7 Oral macrolides and tetracycline derivatives

Both groups of oral antibiotics possess antibacterial and anti-inflammatory properties. The positive effect is reached by the inhibition of collagenase and also by the anti-chemotactic effects, which are believed to improve patients' symptoms by stabilizing the lipid layer of the tear film. This treatment is recommended, especially in chronic blepharitis and MGD along with lid hygiene and warm compresses of various types. MGD is considered to be the main cause of EDE, which is a predominant form of DE responsible for about 70% of cases. Thus, MGD treatment plays a crucial role in DED management.

The treatment regimen for azithromycin seems unified for all clinical studies (500 mg on day 1 and then 250 mg/day for 4 days), while there are significant differences among doxycycline regimens (20–200 mg/day for 2–6 months). Some studies have even proposed the use of a low dose of doxycycline (20 mg) on a long-term basis [30]. Currently, there is no consensus on the unified treatment schedule with doxycycline.

Based on the current knowledge oral macrolide or tetracycline antibiotics are recommended in DED treatment as a "step 2" option recommended by the TFOS DEWS II guidelines [9].

5. Conclusions

Understanding the role of inflammation on the cellular and molecular level may lead to improve treatment options for patients. A new approach to DED treatment should be focused to target not only symptoms but also break the pathological dry eye cycle.

Conflict of interest

None.

DOI: http://dx.doi.org/10.5772/intechopen.114118

Author details

Anna Nowińska[1,2]

1 Clinical Department of Ophthalmology, Faculty of Medical Sciences in Zabrze, Medical University of Silesia, Katowice, Poland

2 Ophthalmology Department, District Railway Hospital, Katowice, Poland

*Address all correspondence to: anna.nowinska@sum.edu.pl

References

[1] Craig JP, Nichols KK, Akpek EK, Caffery B, Dua HS, Joo CK, et al. TFOS DEWS II definition and classification report. The Ocular Surface. 2017;**15**:276-283. DOI: 10.1016/J.JTOS.2017.05.008

[2] Baudouin C. A new approach for better comprehension of diseases of the ocular surface. Journal Français d'Ophtalmologie. 2007;**30**:239-246. DOI: 10.1016/S0181-5512(07)89584-2

[3] Baudouin C, Aragona P, Messmer EM, Tomlinson A, Calonge M, Boboridis KG, et al. Role of hyperosmolarity in the pathogenesis and management of dry eye disease: Proceedings of the OCEAN group meeting. The Ocular Surface. 2013;**11**:246-258. DOI: 10.1016/j.jtos.2013.07.003

[4] Stapleton F, Alves M, Bunya VY, Jalbert I, Lekhanont K, Malet F, et al. TFOS DEWS II epidemiology report. The Ocular Surface. 2017;**15**:334-365. DOI: 10.1016/J.JTOS.2017.05.003

[5] Daniel Nelson J, Shimazaki J, Benitez-del-Castillo JM, Craig J, McCulley JP, Den S, et al. The international workshop on meibomian gland dysfunction: Report of the definition and classification subcommittee. Investigative Ophthalmology & Visual Science. 2011;**52**:1930-1937. DOI: 10.1167/IOVS.10-6997B

[6] Magno MS, Utheim TP, Snieder H, Hammond CJ, Vehof J. The relationship between dry eye and sleep quality. The Ocular Surface. 2021;**20**:13-19. DOI: 10.1016/j.jtos.2020.12.009

[7] Almutairi R, Algezlan S, Bayamin R, Alrumaih S, Almutairi R, Alkahtani R, et al. The association between dry eye and sleep quality among the adult population of Saudi Arabia. Cureus. 2022;**14**:e22736. DOI: 10.7759/cureus.22736

[8] Wolffsohn JS, Arita R, Chalmers R, Djalilian A, Dogru M, Dumbleton K, et al. TFOS DEWS II diagnostic methodology report. The Ocular Surface. 2017;**15**:539-574. DOI: 10.1016/j.jtos.2017.05.001

[9] Jones L, Downie LE, Korb D, Benitez-del-Castillo JM, Dana R, Deng SX, et al. TFOS DEWS II management and therapy report. The Ocular Surface. 2017;**15**:575-628. DOI: 10.1016/j.jtos.2017.05.006

[10] Leonardi A, Modugno RL, Salami E. Allergy and dry eye disease. Ocular Immunology and Inflammation. 2021;**29**:1168-1176. DOI: 10.1080/09273948.2020.1841804

[11] Zemba M, Ionescu MA, Pîrvulescu RA, Dumitrescu OM, Daniel-Constantin B, Radu M, et al. Biomarkers of ocular allergy and dry eye disease. Romanian Journal of Ophthalmology. 2023;**67**:250-259. DOI: 10.22336/rjo.2023.42

[12] Alhatem A, Cavalcanti B, Hamrah P. In vivo confocal microscopy in dry eye disease and related conditions. Seminars in Ophthalmology. 2012;**27**:138-148. DOI: 10.3109/08820538.2012.711416

[13] Villani E, Mantelli F, Nucci P. In-vivo confocal microscopy of the ocular surface. Current Opinion in Allergy and Clinical Immunology. 2013;**13**:569-576. DOI: 10.1097/ACI.0b013e328364ec92

[14] Chen Y, Dana R. Autoimmunity in dry eye disease—An updated review of evidence on effector and memory Th17 cells in disease pathogenicity.

Autoimmunity Reviews. 2021;**20**:102933. DOI: 10.1016/j.autrev.2021.102933

[15] Foulsham W, Mittal SK, Taketani Y, Chen Y, Nakao T, Chauhan SK, et al. Aged mice exhibit severe exacerbations of dry eye disease with an amplified memory Th17 cell response. The American Journal of Pathology. 2020;**190**:1474-1482. DOI: 10.1016/j.ajpath.2020.03.016

[16] Perez VL, Stern ME, Pflugfelder SC. Inflammatory basis for dry eye disease flares. Experimental Eye Research. 2020;**201**:108294. DOI: 10.1016/j.exer.2020.108294

[17] Cha S-H, Lee J-S, Oum B-S, Kim C-D. Corneal epithelial cellular dysfunction from benzalkonium chloride (BAC) in vitro. Clinical & Experimental Ophthalmology. 2004;**32**:180-184. DOI: 10.1111/j.1442-9071.2004.00782.x

[18] Epstein SP, Chen D, Asbell PA. Evaluation of biomarkers of inflammation in response to benzalkonium chloride on corneal and conjunctival epithelial cells. Journal of Ocular Pharmacology and Therapeutics. 2009;**25**:415-424. DOI: 10.1089/jop.2008.0140

[19] Baudouin C. Detrimental effect of preservatives in eyedrops: Implications for the treatment of glaucoma. Acta Ophthalmologica. 2008;**86**:716-726

[20] Jun JH, Bang SP, Park HS, Yoon D, Ahn JY, Kim SJ, et al. A randomized multicenter clinical evaluation of sequential application of 0.3% and 0.15% hyaluronic acid for treatment of dry eye. Japanese Journal of Ophthalmology. 2022;**66**:58-67. DOI: 10.1007/S10384-021-00885-X

[21] Kojima T, Nagata T, Kudo H, Müller-Lierheim WGK, van Setten G-B, Dogru M, et al. The effects of high molecular weight hyaluronic acid eye drop application in environmental dry eye stress model mice. International Journal of Molecular Sciences. 2020;**21**:3516. DOI: 10.3390/ijms21103516

[22] Cejka C, Kossl J, Hermankova B, Holan V, Kubinova S, Olmiere C, et al. The healing of oxidative injuries with trehalose in UVB-irradiated rabbit corneas. Oxidative Medicine and Cellular Longevity. 2019;**2019**:1-10. DOI: 10.1155/2019/1857086

[23] Brar S, Vanga HR, Ganesh S. Comparison of efficacy of trehalose-based eye drops versus topical 0.1% hyaluronic acid for Management of clinically significant dry eye using non-invasive investigational modalities. International Ophthalmology. 2021;**41**:3349-3359. DOI: 10.1007/s10792-021-01897-9

[24] Panigrahi T, Shivakumar S, Shetty R, D'souza S, Nelson EJR, Sethu S, et al. Trehalose augments autophagy to mitigate stress induced inflammation in human corneal cells. The Ocular Surface. 2019;**17**:699-713. DOI: 10.1016/j.jtos.2019.08.004

[25] Cagini C, Di Lascio G, Torroni G, Mariniello M, Meschini G, Lupidi M, et al. Dry eye and inflammation of the ocular surface after cataract surgery: Effectiveness of a tear film substitute based on trehalose/hyaluronic acid vs hyaluronic acid to resolve signs and symptoms. Journal of Cataract and Refractive Surgery. 2021;**47**:1430-1435. DOI: 10.1097/j.jcrs.0000000000000652

[26] Cagini C, Torroni G, Mariniello M, Di Lascio G, Martone G, Balestrazzi A. Trehalose/sodium hyaluronate eye drops in post-cataract ocular surface disorders. International Ophthalmology. 2021;**41**:3065-3071. DOI: 10.1007/s10792-021-01869-z

[27] Eghtedari Y, Oh LJ, Girolamo N, Watson SL. The role of topical N-acetylcysteine in ocular therapeutics. Survey of Ophthalmology. 2022;**67**:608-622. DOI: 10.1016/j.survophthal.2021.07.008

[28] Prinz J, Maffulli N, Fuest M, Walter P, Bell A, Migliorini F. Efficacy of topical administration of corticosteroids for the management of dry eye disease: Systematic review and meta-analysis. Life. 1932;**2022**:12. DOI: 10.3390/life12111932

[29] Liu S-H, Saldanha IJ, Abraham AG, Rittiphairoj T, Hauswirth S, Gregory D, et al. Topical corticosteroids for dry eye. Cochrane Database of Systematic Reviews. 21 Oct 2022;**10**(10):CD015070. DOI: 10.1002/14651858.CD015070.pub2

[30] Yoo S-E, Lee D-C, Chang M-H. The effect of low-dose doxycycline therapy in chronic meibomian gland dysfunction. Korean Journal of Ophthalmology. 2005;**19**:258. DOI: 10.3341/kjo.2005.19.4.258

Section 3

Miscellaneous

Chapter 6

Challenges of the Intraocular Pressure Measurements in the Keratitis

Cansu Yuksel Elgin

Abstract

The maintenance of the aqueous humor circulation is vital for nourishing the anterior segment structures and maintaining the shape of the eyeball. Imbalances in the production and drainage of aqueous humor are well-known occurrences during inflammatory processes in the anterior chamber, with keratitis being a major contributor. Elevated intraocular pressure (IOP) is a common complication during active microbial keratitis. However, even under normal conditions, corneal biomechanical properties, thickness, and curvature can complicate the accuracy of IOP measurements. Ongoing research is exploring the relationship between corneal characteristics and IOP. Corneal conditions related to keratitis, such as band-keratopathy, corneal edema, astigmatism, and corneal ectatic disorders, pose significant challenges for managing high-pressure-related complications. Different IOP measurement techniques may be preferable in various corneal prominent conditions. Regular IOP checks are necessary to avoid possible optic nerve damage during keratitis treatment. It is crucial to select the appropriate measurement technique and consider potential over- and underestimations of IOP due to corneal disorders.

Keywords: keratitis, intraocular pressure, pressure measurement, corneal disorders, cornea

1. Introduction

Intraocular pressure (IOP), which refers to the internal pressure of the eye, is a measure of the fluid pressure inside the eye. However, it is not practically feasible to directly measure the pressure inside the eye in routine clinical practice. Therefore, all clinical methods of measuring IOP are based on estimating it through the external surface of the eye. None of these methods are precise enough to accurately measure the true IOP using invasive techniques. Even the Goldmann applanation tonometer (GAT), which is commonly accepted as the current gold standard tonometer, cannot consistently provide reliable measurements in all conditions. The fundamental principle of applanation tonometry is based on the Imbert–Fick law, which can be expressed by the equation: Intraocular pressure = Contact force/Area of contact. However, this formula would work accurately only if the cornea were infinitely thin, perfectly elastic, and flexible, which is not the case. The measurement of IOP using

GAT can be influenced by factors such as corneal thickness, curvature, modulus of elasticity, rigidity, and tear film. In particular, if there are ocular surface pathologies present, these corneal parameters are affected, leading to compromised accuracy in IOP measurements.

IOP is a critical parameter in the diagnosis and management of ocular diseases, including keratitis. However, obtaining accurate IOP measurements in patients with keratitis can be challenging due to several factors. In this paper, we review the challenges associated with IOP measurements in keratitis, including the effects of corneal thinning and scarring, tear film instability, and the use of topical medications. We also discuss various methods for measuring IOP in keratitis patients, including GAT, Tono-Pen, dynamic contour tonometer, the rebound tonometer, the ocular response analyzer, and their limitations. Finally, we suggest strategies for overcoming these challenges and improving IOP measurements in keratitis patients.

2. Keratitis-related conditions affecting the IOP measurement

Keratitis is an inflammatory condition that affects the cornea, the transparent outer layer of the eye. It can be caused by infectious agents such as bacteria, fungi, or viruses, or by noninfectious factors such as trauma, contact lens wear, or autoimmune disorders. Keratitis can lead to a different range of corneal thickness differences from thinning–scarring to thickening, edema, and calcification which can affect the accuracy of intraocular pressure (IOP) measurements, a critical parameter in the diagnosis and management of ocular diseases, including keratitis.

Corneal thinning and scarring can affect the accuracy of IOP measurements as they can lead to a reduction in corneal rigidity, which can cause underestimation of IOP. Several studies have shown that IOP measurements in keratitis patients are lower than in normal subjects due to corneal thinning and scarring [1, 2]. In addition, corneal infiltrates, or subepithelial calcium hydroxyapatite deposition named band-keratopathy, can increase the thickness and rigidity of the cornea, leading to overestimation of IOP [3]. The Ocular Hypertension Treatment Study (OHTS) found that cornea thickness is a major determinant in the glaucomatous process. At first sight, all the thickening and thinning process of the cornea seems like the effect of central corneal thickness (CCT) on IOP measurements. But the effect of the keratitis not only affect the CCT but also affect corneal curvature, modulus of elasticity – rigidity and tear film. The range of cornea's biomechanical properties, like energy absorption and resistance of the deformation, which influences its capacity to dampen fluctuations in IOP, may influence tonometry. For example, the edema may cause CCT thickening but also may bring resistance deficiency. So at some points, you may get under-estimated IOP values even in the thickened corneas. Consequently, throughout the progression of keratitis, these parameters are often interconnected and complex, emphasizing the need to consider them during clinical evaluation.

Besides the cornea-related parameters, tear film instability is another challenge in IOP measurements in keratitis patients. Tear film instability can lead to fluctuations in IOP measurements due to changes in tear volume and composition. Several studies have reported that tear film instability can affect the accuracy of IOP measurements obtained using GAT, the most commonly used method for measuring IOP [4, 5]. However, the effects of tear film can be avoided by dynamic contour tonometry, rebound tonometer, noncontact tonometry [6, 7].

DOI: http://dx.doi.org/10.5772/intechopen.112417

The other independent factor from cornea is topical medications. Topical medications used for the treatment of keratitis can affect IOP measurements by altering the corneal properties. Although ophthalmic steroids can cause steroid-induced high intraocular pressure, several studies have shown that topical steroids can reduce corneal rigidity and lead to underestimation of IOP [8, 9]. Similarly, topical antibiotics can affect corneal thickness and rigidity, leading to inaccurate IOP measurements [10].

After taking account of these keratitis-related conditions, we will evaluate the different IOP measurement principles with their pros and cons.

3. Methods for measuring IOP in keratitis patients

3.1 Applanation tonometries

Goldmann applanation tonometry (GAT) (see **Figure 1**) is the leading method of the applanation tonometries and is widely accepted as the gold standard for IOP measurement. However, it has several limitations in keratitis patients. It requires a clear cornea for accurate measurements, which is not always possible in keratitis patients with corneal edema, scarring, or astigmatism. In addition, GAT measurements can be affected by tear film instability, as mentioned earlier. Also, if there are coexisting eye lid scarring-retraction pathologies, this will lead to overestimation of the IOP measurement. The CCT is considered as the most important parameter in the GAT measurements, and many studies address this problem by proposing a number of correction formulas. Although CCT may give information about the estimation of the real IOP, the CCT-based correction formula is not advised to be

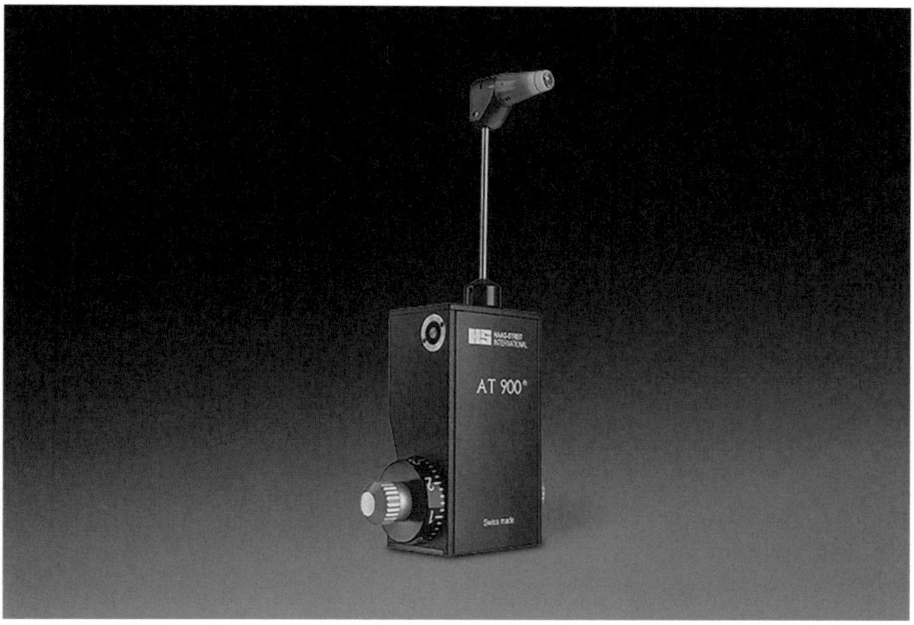

Figure 1.
Goldmann applanation tonometry.

applied to individuals [11, 12]. The other limitations of this technique are the risk of contamination and the pulsatile changes in the measurements.

There are also noncontact types of applanation tonometers that eliminate contamination risks. One of them is *air-puff tonometer* (**Figure 2a**). Air-puff tonometers employ a rapid and controlled puff of air to applanate the cornea and measure IOP. They offer several advantages over traditional methods, including noninvasiveness, patient comfort, and rapid measurements. As for the first property, air-puff tonometers do not require any physical contact with the cornea, reducing the risk of infection and injury. For patient comfort, these tonometers eliminate the need for topical anesthetic eye drops and the discomfort associated with corneal contact. Finally, for rapid measurements, air-puff tonometers provide quick IOP readings, making them suitable for large-scale screenings and busy clinical settings. However, limitations exist with air-puff tonometry, including potential variability in measurements due to factors such as corneal thickness, ocular surface irregularities, and patient cooperation. Also, its measurements are brand-dependent and less accurate than the GAT's. Mostly, it underestimates IOP at high ranges and overestimates IOP at low ranges as compared to the GAT.

In this device, air-puff applanating force, flattens the cornea, and this force is covered to the mmHg. As it is expected, corneal infiltrations, deformations, and irregularities may lead to resistance or softening on the applanation force, and in consequence, this might lead to under or over-estimation of the IOP.

The other noncontact type of applanation tonometer is *ocular response analyzer* (**Figure 2b**). It also applanates the cornea by air-puff, but the air column continues to emit with increasing intensity until the cornea is indented. Then the force of the air column decreases until the cornea is once again at a point of applanation. The difference in the pressures at the two applanation points is a measure of the corneal biomechanic properties (rigidity or floppiness). When confronting the unusual cornea, it helps us to think about corneal biomechanics to accurately assess IOP and glaucoma risk. Mathematical equations are used to "correct" the applanation point for high or

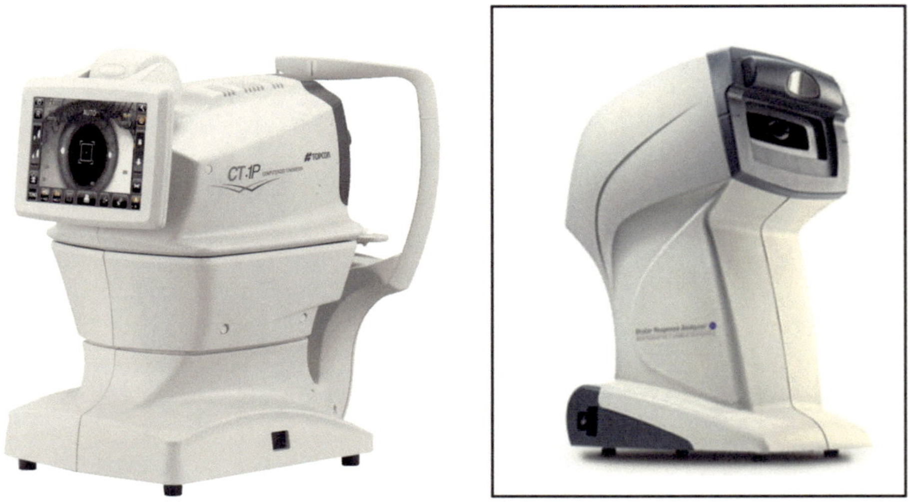

(a) (b)

Figure 2.
Air-puff tonometer and ocular response analyzer.

low elasticity. This "corrected" IOP is thought to be less dependent on corneal thickness than other forms of applanated pressures [13].

3.2 Indentation tonometers

The principle of indentation tonometry is that a force or a weight will indent an eye surface by way of the transducer to detect the transmitted pressure. The prototype of the indentation tonometers is the Schiøtz tonometer which was introduced many years ago and is no longer currently used.

The *Tono-Pen* (**Figure 3**) is the current form of the indentation tonometers. Indeed, the Tono-Pen involves both applanation and indentation processes, and it works both process calculations in multiple measurements. It is a small, handheld, battery-powered portable device and brings many advantages at some points. The main advantages of the Tono-Pen are its portability, not requiring a slit-lamp, or electricity, and its measurement ability in both supine and upright positions. A disposable latex cap is used for each patient, which helps to reduce the risk of infection between patients. More than that, Tono-Pen comes into prominence, especially in patients with eye scarring or irregular corneas like keratitis. Its measurements are well-correlated with Goldmann tonometry within normal IOP ranges. Moreover, it provides better accuracy in edematous corneas than GAT and dynamic contour tonometry [14]. But, Tono-pen was found to consistently underestimate IOP, with a significant error for IOP values >30 mmHg; also Tono-Pen can be significantly affected by CCT.

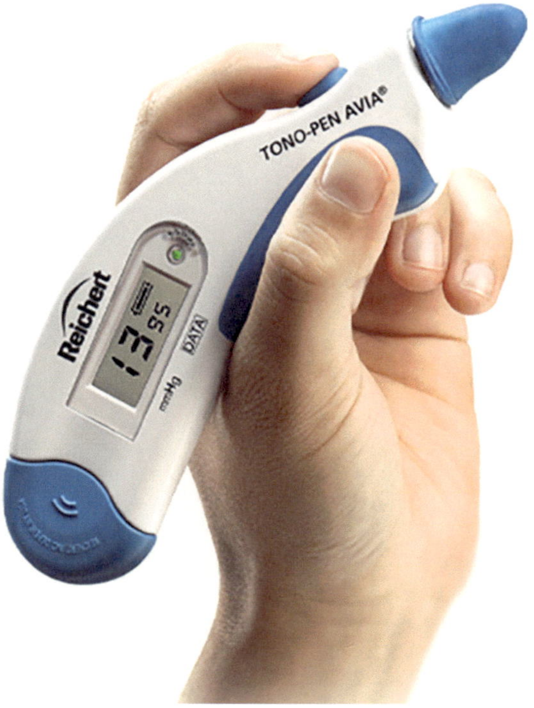

Figure 3.
Tono-Pen.

3.3 Rebound tonometry

Rebound tonometry has emerged as a noninvasive and reliable method for assessing IOP. They are the last generated tonometer models but are well-accepted and widely used devices worldwide (**Figure 4**). Like Tono-pen, it is portable, fast, and easy to use and does not need a slit-lamp or electricity. Its 1.8 mm diameter subtle probe impacts onto the cornea and then rebounds from the eye with a different velocity, which varies according to the IOP. Its small surface contact makes it suitable for measuring damaged corneas. Also, the subtle probe may be less traumatic on the cornea than GAT, and it could offer a better alternative in keratitis patients to provide information regarding IOP. Subtle probe contact leads to minimal discomfort during the procedure, making it suitable for individuals who may be sensitive or anxious about eye examinations. Rebound tonometers are portable and easy to operate, making them suitable for use in various clinical settings. The simplicity of the technique allows healthcare professionals to quickly and accurately measure IOP, facilitating screening programs and enabling frequent monitoring of patients with glaucoma. Moreover, it also has a high degree of versatility and reliability. Rebound tonometry provides accurate IOP measurements across a wide range of corneal conditions and shapes. It is less influenced by corneal thickness and biomechanical properties, factors that can affect other tonometry methods. This versatility ensures more reliable and consistent IOP readings, enhancing the diagnosis, treatment, and management of ocular conditions. IOP measurements obtained with this device have also been shown to be influenced by CCT with higher IOP readings with thicker corneas. Also, it is affected by other biomechanical properties of the cornea, including corneal hysteresis and corneal resistance factor.

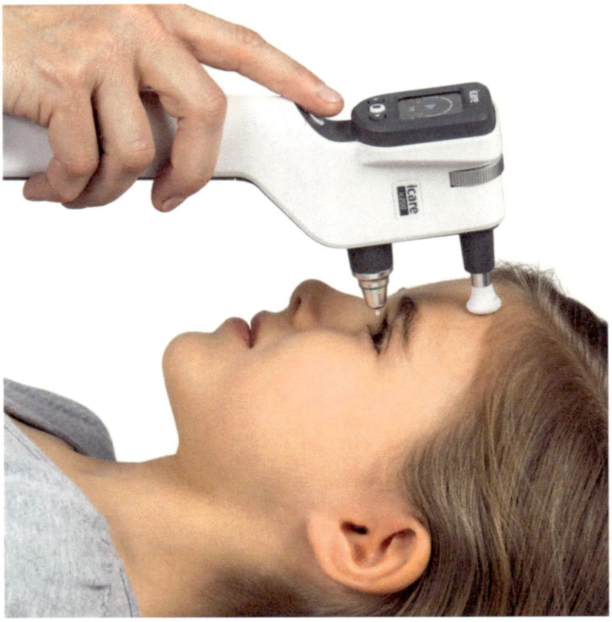

Figure 4.
Rebound tonometry.

3.4 Dynamic contour tonometry (DCT)

DCT is a method of tonometry that measures IOP by detecting changes in the contour of the cornea. It works according to the Pascal principle which the pressure changes applied to the wall surface of a fluid in a contained enclosed place. DCT utilizes a sensor tip to detect changes in the ocular pulse waveform, enabling accurate IOP assessment. It takes about 8–10 sec corneal contact in order to provide IOP measurement. The advantages of DCT include accuracy and reproducibility as it accounts for corneal biomechanical properties and ocular pulsations, leading to more precise IOP measurements compared to traditional methods. Ocular pulse amplitude (OPA) measurement provides indirect information about choroid perfusion and also the eradication of the pulsatile changes on IOP. Several studies have shown that DCT is a reliable method for measuring IOP in keratitis patients [15–17]. Although reduced accuracy in the presence of irregular corneas, DCT is also applicable to various corneal conditions and shapes, making it suitable for a diverse range of patients. Nevertheless, DCT also has limitations, including difficulties, such as the need for a slit-lamp, topical anesthetic, longer corneal contact in a good head and eye position, trained staff, and highly cooperative patients.

Table 1 summarizes frequently-used IOP measurement tonometers and presents their advantages and disadvantages.

3.5 Digital palpation

After familiarizing with various instruments produced through different principles of physics, which possess numerous advantages and weaknesses, it is possible that none of these devices may be effective in certain exceptional circumstances. In cases of severe eye pain and sensitivity, suspicion of globe rupture, indications of severe infection, and specific situations where sufficient lid aperture cannot be achieved, it may be necessary to perform intraocular pressure estimation using fingertip. Making a comparison with the patient's unaffected eye in these situations can facilitate the estimation process.

4. Strategies for overcoming challenges in IOP measurements in keratitis patients

To overcome the challenges associated with IOP measurements in keratitis patients, several strategies can be employed. These include corneal pachymetry, tear film stabilization, and the management of topical medications.

Corneal pachymetry is a noninvasive method for measuring corneal thickness, which can help to correct IOP measurements in patients with corneal edema or thinning. Corneal pachymetry can be used to adjust IOP measurements obtained using GAT or as a baseline for measurements obtained using DCT.

Tear film stabilization can be achieved through artificial tears or punctual plugs, reducing fluctuations in IOP measurements due to tear film instability.

The management of topical medications in keratitis patients can help to reduce the effects of these medications on IOP measurements. This can include reducing the frequency or dose of medications that affect corneal properties or switching to alternative medications that have less impact on IOP measurements.

	Advantages	Disadvantages
GAT	Widely accepted gold standard technique	7.35 mm2 contact area by truncated conic probe
	Designed by basic physic principle, Imbert–Fick law: P = F/S	Topical anesthesia and fluorescein drop
		contamination and cornea damage risk
		Upright position on a slit-lamp
		Influenced by the CCT, tear film, cornea biomechanics
		Subjective measurement
Air -Puff Tonometer	No need to touch the cornea	Influenced by corneal parameters (CCT-biomechanics-edema)
	Designed by the measurement of the air force of corneal flattening	Slit-lamp positioning
	Objective measurements (can be taken by nonmedical staff)	Ideal as a screening (less accurate than GAT)
	Reduced risk of infection and injury	
Ocular Response Analyzer	No need to touch the cornea	Relatively expensive device
	Designed by the measurement of the air force inward and outward applanation of the cornea	Not extensive usage
	Capable of measuring corneal biomechanics (electro-optical system monitor the deformation of the cornea)	Slit-lamp positioning
	Corrected IOP calculation (less dependent measurements by corneal parameters-(CCT-biomechanics-edema))	
	Objective measurements (can be taken by nonmedical staff)	
	Reduced risk of infection and injury	
Tono-Pen	Portable lightweight, handheld, battery-powered device	Contact method and cornea damage risk
	Principles of applanation and indentation-	Significantly affected by CCT
	Disposable latex cap – reduced risk of infection	Significant error for high IOP values
	Measurement in both supine and upright positions.	Intra-session repeated measurements' variabilities are found high
	Better accuracy in edematous corneas	Significant variations from GAT
Rebound Tonometry	Widespread accepted and used device in a short exposed time	Influenced by the CCT, tear film, cornea biomechanics
	Designed by the rebound subtle probe's velocity, which impacts the cornea	Influenced by peripheral corneal measurements
	Portable lightweight, handheld, battery-powered device	Underestimation IOP at a higher level

	Advantages	Disadvantages
	Measurement in both supine and upright positions (last version)	
	Small surface contact-less traumatic compared to GAT and provides measurement across the irregular cornea	
	Excellent repeatability and good reliability (especially for normal range)	
DCT	Designed by measurement of the dynamic pressure changes in a fluid-enclosed space	Need for a slit-lamp–topical anesthesia
	Detection of the dynamic pulsatile fluctuations and ocular pulse amplitude	Need for trained staff and highly cooperative patients
	Contour matching principle between cornea and tip – theoretically elimination of the corneal parameters	Long contact time (at least 8 s)-difficult to use
	Less influenced method by the properties of the cornea	Reduced accuracy in the irregular corneas
	Disposable sensor caps in order to avoid the risk of infection	

Table 1.
Advantages and disadvantages of different IOP measurement techniques.

5. Conclusion

IOP measurements are critical in the diagnosis and management of ocular diseases, including keratitis. However, obtaining accurate IOP measurements in keratitis patients can be challenging due to several factors, including corneal thinning and scarring, tear film instability, and the use of topical medications. Various methods of tonometry, have been proposed as alternatives to GAT in keratitis patients, but their accuracy in this population has still limitations, and they are still under investigation. Strategies for overcoming these challenges, such as corneal pachymetry, tear film stabilization, and topical medication management, can help to improve the accuracy of IOP measurements in keratitis patients.

Acknowledgements

There is no funding to be declared.

Conflict of interest

The author declares no conflict of interest.

Author details

Cansu Yuksel Elgin
Istanbul University-Cerrahpasa, Turkey

*Address all correspondence to: cansu.elgin@iuc.edu.tr

References

[1] Jadidi K, Mohazzab-Torabi S, Pirhadi S, Naderi M, Yekta A, Sardari S, et al. A study of corneal biomechanics in delayed-onset mustard gas keratopathy compared to cases with corneal scarring and normal corneas. Eye & Contact Lens. 1 Mar 2019;**45**(2):112-116

[2] Kaufman SC. Anterior segment complications of herpes zoster ophthalmicus. Ophthalmology. 1 Feb 2008;**115**(2):S24-S32

[3] Tham YC, Li X, Wong TY, Quigley HA, Aung T, Cheng CY. Global prevalence of glaucoma and projections of glaucoma burden through 2040: A systematic review and meta-analysis. Ophthalmology. 2014;**121**(11):2081-2090

[4] Kim YK, Ha SW, Kim CY. The effects of tear film on Goldmann applanation tonometry and dynamic contour tonometry. Korean Journal of Ophthalmology. 2009;**23**(4):254-257

[5] Hsu SY, Sheu MM, Hsu AH, Wu KY, Yeh JI, Tien JN, et al. Comparisons of intraocular pressure measurements: Goldmann applanation tonometry, noncontact tonometry, Tono-Pen tonometry, and dynamic contour tonometry. Eye. Jul 2009;**23**(7):1582-1588

[6] Clemen CI, Parker DGA, Goldberg I. Intra-ocular pressure measurement in a patient with a thin, thick or abnormal cornea. Open Ophthalmological Journal. 2016;**10**:35-43

[7] Chiara E. Assessment of true intraocular pressure: The gap between theory and practical data. Survey of Ophthalmology. 2008;**53**(3):203-218

[8] Prata TS, Sousa AM, Melo LA Jr. Influence of topical corticosteroids on the biomechanical behavior of the cornea. Arquivos Brasileiros de Oftalmologia. 2010;**73**(3):235-239

[9] Sihota R, Dada T, Gupta V, et al. Evaluation of the effect of topical application of corticosteroids on the biomechanical properties of the cornea. Eye (London, England). 2008;**22**(7)

[10] Kouchaki B, Hashemi H, Yekta A. Comparison of current tonometry techniques in measurement of intraocular pressure. Journal of Current Ophthalmology. 1 Jun 2017;**29**(2):92-97

[11] Park J, Cho HS, Moon JI. Comparison of intraocular pressure measurements obtained by dynamic contour tonometry and Goldmann applanation tonometry in children. Korean Journal of Ophthalmology. 2015;**29**(5):332-337

[12] Park SJ, Ang GS, Nicholas S, Wells AP. The effect of thin, thick, and normal corneas on Goldmann intraocular pressure measurements and correction formulae in individual eyes. Ophthalmology. 2012;**119**(3):443-449. DOI: 10.1016/j.ophtha.2011.07.058

[13] Stamper R. A history of intraocular pressure and its measurement. Optometry and Vision Science. 2011;**88**(1):E16-E28

[14] Kontadakis GA, Pennos A, Pentari I, Kymionis GD, Pallikaris IG, Ginis H. Accuracy of dynamic contour tonometry, Goldmann applanation tonometry, and Tono-Pen XL in edematous corneas. Therapeutic Advance in. Ophthalmology. 2020;**2020**:12. DOI: 10.1177/2515841420923190

[15] Copt RP, Thomas R, Mermoud A. Corneal thickness in ocular

hypertension, primary open-angle glaucoma, and normal tension glaucoma. Archives of Ophthalmology. 1999;**117**(1):14-16

[16] Bochmann F, Kaufmann C, Thiel MA. Dynamic contour tonometry versus Goldmann applanation tonometry: Challenging the gold standard. Expert Review of Ophthalmology. 1 Dec 2010;**5**(6):743-749

[17] Realini T, Weinreb RN, Hobbs G. Correlation of intraocular pressure measured with Goldmann and dynamic contour tonometry in normal and glaucomatous eyes. Journal of Glaucoma. Feb 2009;**18**(2):119

Chapter 7

Prevention of Corneal Injury in Critically Ill Sedated and Mechanically Ventilated Patients: Theoretical and Evidence-Based Practice

Patricia R. do Prado and Fernanda R.E. Gimenes

Abstract

Any prolonged loss of consciousness due to sedation in critically ill patients may result in eye injuries which may go unnoticed as the patient cannot express his/her reduced vision or pain. Loss of blinking movement and eyelid malocclusion can cause some eye injuries as keratopathies and ulcers, which are the most common eye injuries in these patients. In at-risk patients (intubated and ventilated), screening for corneal injuries should be carried out using a fluorescein test. Protection of the cornea depends on its moisturization, which itself depends on eyelid closure, blinking, and the quality of the aqueous film present on the cornea. These protective components are regularly reduced in critically ill patients. Some cohort studies indicate that the peak incidence of corneal injuries occurs after first-week admission in critically ill patients. In intubated and ventilated patients, an eye gel and polyethylene chamber are the most effective interventions to prevent corneal injuries.

Keywords: corneal injury, intensive care units, nursing care, prevention and control, mechanically ventilated patients

1. Introduction

Currently, more than 10 million people in the world are affected by eye diseases that can result in irreversible corneal injuries. In critically ill sedated and intubated) patients, who often fail to notify nurses of possible eye problems, assessment, prevention, and treatment of eye injuries are imperative [1–3].

The cornea is the anterior structure of the eye through which ultraviolet rays enter and is responsible for refraction, focusing the rays on the retina to provide adequate vision. The cornea has five distinct layers: epithelium, Bowman's layer, stroma, Descemet's membrane, and endothelium. The epithelium is the first layer of the cornea and contains superficial nerves to protect and regenerate the eye. Next, there is the Bowman layer/membrane, which is very resistant and has the main function of serving as a barrier against microorganisms. The stroma is the most consistent layer of the cornea, occupying 90% of its thickness. Descemet's membrane is resistant to the penetration of microorganisms and gets thicker over the years. The endothelium is the innermost layer of the cornea and has the function of hydrating the eyes [4, 5].

To maintain a healthy cornea and good vision, each layer must function properly [1, 4]. The proper functioning of these layers also depends on the blinking and closing mechanisms of the eyelids, which provide corneal lubrication and protection, respectively [1, 6–8].

In critically ill patients using sedatives, muscle blockers, and mechanical ventilation, the protective mechanisms of the corneas are altered and do not provide blink and close eyelids reflex whose corneas are exposed and may present with dryness, exposure keratitis, and ulcers which result in temporary or permanent loss of vision [8–12].

In this chapter, we will address the main corneal injuries, risk factors, and interventions to prevent corneal injuries in critically ill patients.

2. Epidemiology, definition, and prevention of corneal injuries

2.1 Corneal injuries: Incidence

The incidence of corneal injury in sedated and ventilated critically ill patients ranges from 2.6 to 60.0%. According to previous studies, the incidence of corneal injury is lower in units that have eye care protocols implemented and nursing training to prevent the event. However, evidence-based practices are still incipient [2, 13–15]. Developing and implementing continuing education programs for promoting eye care knowledge, attitude, and practice are strongly recommended [2, 16, 17].

Several prospective cohort and clinical-randomized studies evaluated the occurrence of corneal injury in adult ICU patients. In India, incidences of 13.2% [18] and 21.0% [19] were identified in 5 days of follow-up. In Iran, also on day 5 follow-up, 32.2% had dry eye disease (DED) and 13.8% developed corneal injury [13]. In Jordan, 57% had exposure keratopathy [20].

In Brazil, incidences of 16.3% were identified in Acre [9], 20.0% in Rio de Janeiro [10], and 59.4% in Minas Gerais [21], respectively. The difference in the incidence of corneal injury in critically ill patients in the same country can be explained by the characteristics of the patients (percentage of sedated patients, on mechanical ventilation, with corneal exposure, autoimmune diseases, and diabetes, for example) that may contribute to an increased risk of corneal injury. Nevertheless, the climate and relative humidity characteristics have never been evaluated in studies, although the literature has already shown the causality between lower humidity and greater risk for DED and corneal injury, a fact that should be considered in future research [22, 23].

In Minas Gerais, Brazil [21], where the incidence of injury was 59.4%, the prevalence of patients on mechanical ventilation was higher, 78.7% against 58.3% in Rio de Janeiro (Santos et al., 2023) and 64.2% in Acre [8]. Still, in Minas Gerais, the climate is equatorial and dry in winter, with a relative humidity of around 20%. In the states of Rio de Janeiro and Acre, the climates are tropical maritime hot and humid, and tropical humid, with humidity around 80%, respectively, which can also interfere with the incidence of corneal injury [22, 23].

In addition, the incidence of corneal injury is lower in critically ill pediatric patients due to shorter mechanical ventilation time and lower occurrence of chemosis (conjunctival edema). In the United States, an incidence of 19% of corneal injury in children and 60% in critically ill adults was identified [24].

The main changes in the corneas are dry eye disease, exposure keratitis, and corneal ulcers, which will be discussed below.

2.2 Corneal injuries definition

The ICU is an environment predisposing to the development of dry eye disease and, consequently, corneal injuries [8, 25–27].

Dry eye disease occurs due to impaired tear film production or increased evaporation. In ICU patients, the tear film is compromised due to disorder in the mechanisms responsible for ocular lubrication and protection. This occurs due to the use of sedative drugs and muscle relaxants that prevent blinking and closing the eyelids [8, 25–27].

Also, mechanical ventilation with high end-expiratory pressure (PEEP) and orotracheal tube with strong fixation contribute to the appearance of conjunctival edema and chemosis. Chemosis impairs eyelid closure and causes lagophthalmos [6–9, 12, 25–28].

In addition to the patient's intrinsic problems, the ICU is a unit with air conditioning which favors greater evaporation of the tear film. Still, there are many microorganisms that can colonize the cornea causing fungal or viral keratitis or ulcers, for example. Critically ill patients receive many interventions, which can accidentally injure the patient's corneas during airway aspiration, prone positioning, bed bath, and changing central access dressings or orotracheal tube [1, 6, 7, 12, 25, 28].

Therefore, in patients who do not blink and close their eyes properly, the corneas are vulnerable to ocular dryness which is the first stage of corneal injury. If there are no interventions for this condition, the patient may develop exposure keratitis and corneal ulcers that can cause temporary or permanent loss of vision [1, 7, 12, 25, 26, 28].

Figure 1 shows the pathophysiology of corneal injury in critically ill patients.

2.2.1 Dry eye disease

Dry eye disease (DED) is a multifactorial disease characterized by loss of tear film homeostasis and accompanied by ocular symptoms, in which tear film instability and hyperosmolarity, ocular surface inflammation and damage, and neurosensory abnormalities play etiological roles [25].

The main causes, in sedated and mechanically ventilated patients, are lack of lubrication due to loss of blinking movement, incomplete eyelids closure, which exposes the corneas, environment with low humidity due to the use of air conditioning, invasive interventions, which can lead to corneal trauma and lacerations, and prone positioning. In addition to these factors, patients with autoimmune diseases such as lupus erythematosus and myasthenia gravis, diabetes, and those with chronic ocular graft-versus-host disease have altered tear production. Besides, patients with vitamin A and omega 3 deficiency seem to be more susceptible to dry eye disease [22, 23, 25, 27, 29–33].

Another risk factors for DED include drugs associated with the induction of tear deficiency such as benzodiazepines, oral contraceptives, beta-blockers, hydrochlorothiazide, antiarrhythmics, anticholinergics, antihistamines, decongestants, tricyclic antidepressants, monoamine oxidase inhibitors, antineoplastics, antiparkinsonians, antidiarrheals, thiabendazole, and retinoids [7, 23, 33].

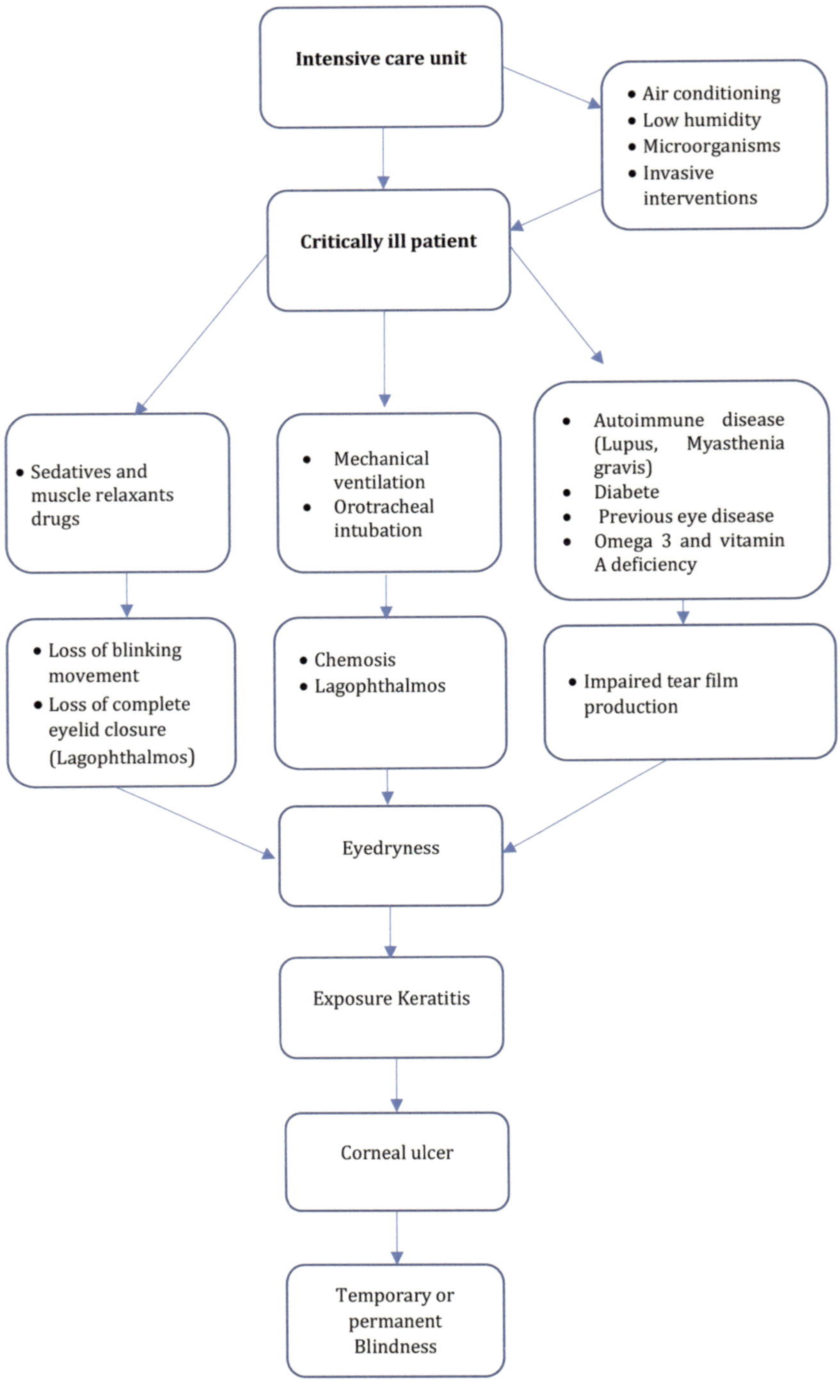

Figure 1.
Pathophysiology of corneal injury in critically ill patients.

The main signs and symptoms of DED are reddish and dull conjunctiva, feeling that there is a foreign body in the eye such as a speck or small particles of dust, burning, itching, ocular discharge, and blurred vision [1, 7, 23, 26, 33].

DED confers inflammation and infections that make the cornea opaque and can lead to vision loss. Thus, patients with DED need to receive lubrication and ocular protection.

2.2.2 Keratitis

"Keratitis is a clinical entity in which inflammatory cells infiltrate different layers of the cornea in response to noxious stimuli from exogenous infectious agents or autoantigens. The inflammatory reaction can result in suppurative fusion of the corneal epithelium and stroma, resulting in the formation of ulcers. This not only results in loss of corneal clarity but also threatens the integrity of the globe and can result in blindness." It is necessary to identify the etiologic agent based on clinical features and appropriate diagnostic tests and to manage these patients with the latest treatment options [27].

In addition to dry eye disease, other causes should be investigated, such as herpes simplex virus type I, bacteria, viruses or fungi infections, ocular trauma caused by equipment or prone positioning, vitamin A and omega 3 deficiency, allergy or sensitivity to cosmetics, and environmental pollution [1, 7, 31, 34, 35].

The main signs and symptoms of keratitis are redness conjunctiva, eye pain, photophobia (sensitivity to light), burning, and blurred vision. The diagnosis of keratitis and corneal ulcer requires confirmation by examining stained smears of corneal scrapings and laboratory cultures of these scrapings.

When it is used, an ophthalmoscope with cobalt blue light and the instillation of fluorescein eye drops pits are visualized on the cornea due to the fluorescein effect and its intensity depends on the severity of the keratitis [1, 6, 7, 31, 34, 35].

2.2.3 Corneal ulcer

A corneal ulcer is one of the presentations of keratitis. It is an ocular emergency characterized by the destruction of epithelial cells secondary to inflammation and necrosis of the corneal stroma. The ulcer appears as a white or grayish spot in the eye that, if left untreated, can lead to blindness. The main causes are lagophthalmos, which causes DED, bacteria, viruses, fungi, amebae, and abrasions/traumas [1, 6, 7, 36, 37].

The main manifestations are conjunctival hyperemia, photophobia, pain, and severe visual disturbances. Diagnosis is performed by the instillation of fluorescein eye drops and visualization through an ophthalmoscope with cobalt light. Microscopic examination of scrapings can identify Acanthamoeba [7, 11, 37].

Treatment will involve the instillation of antibiotic, antifungal, anti-inflammatory, and corticoid eye drops depending on the identified cause [8, 38]. In some cases, surgery and/or corneal transplantation is required to remove the cloudy cornea and replace it with a healthy, transparent cornea [36, 37].

Critical patients are more vulnerable to corneal injury due to changes in the protective mechanisms of the corneas. The prevention of this type of injury depends on the daily assessment by the nursing team, especially in patients with a lowered level of consciousness, using sedative drugs and neuromuscular blockers. In those patients, eye lubrication and protection are recommended [3].

2.3 Corneal injuries: risk factors

The main risk factors for the development of corneal injuries in sedated and ventilated critically patients are mechanical ventilation, sedatives, lagophthalmos, chemosis, and hospitalization for more than 7 days [8–10, 12, 20, 21, 24, 38].

Patients on mechanical ventilation had a chance (ODDS) between 37.8 [10] and 117 [21] times to develop a corneal injury compared to non-ventilated patients.

Patients with lagophthalmos had between 13.4 [10] and 17.15 [8] higher risk (hazard ratio) for corneal injury compared to those without lagophthalmos. In addition, patients with chemosis had between 7.39 [8] and 25 times more chance of presenting the event [10]compared to those who did not have chemosis.

Hospitalization longer than 7 days is also a higher risk factor for the development of corneal injury in critically ill patients (OR: 11.96; 95% CI: 3.27–43.66) [8]. Thus, research involving the assessment of corneal injury should be carried out with a minimum follow-up of 7 days [8, 9, 21, 24].

2.4 Prevention of corneal injuries

The high incidence rate of corneal injury in sedated and mechanically ventilated patients reflects that eye care has been neglected by the health team. This occurs due to the lack of knowledge and attitude of nurses and the absence of patient complaints about dryness and visual discomfort that can culminate in temporary or permanent loss of vision, with preventable adverse events [15, 38–40].

Many interventions have been tested in randomized clinical trials, and recent systematic reviews recommend that eye gel and a polyethylene chamber are the most effective interventions to prevent corneal injury [3, 41–45].

The polyethylene chamber has already been tested in several international and national studies. It has a low cost, is easy to handle, has greater durability, and demonstrated higher effectiveness when compared to eye drops [38, 45]. In addition, the intervention does not require a medical prescription. Studies conducted in Brazil [21], Australia [44, 46], Turkey [47], and Iran [41, 43] demonstrated the effectiveness of the polyethylene chamber; however, the researchers used handmade chambers. Accordingly, it is necessary to create and assess the effectiveness of a polyethylene chamber specifically designed to prevent corneal injury in sedated and mechanically ventilated patients.

The prevention of corneal injury consists primary of ocular lubrication, preferably with gel or ointment eye, and protection of the corneas with a polyethylene chamber for critically ill patients with compromised blinking and closing eye mechanisms. As a recommendation, we suggest that nurses develop an eye care protocol, including eye gel lubrication, for 4 or 6 hours, and a polyethylene chamber, for 12 hours, for sedated mechanically ventilated critically ill patients. In addition, a polyethylene chamber must be commercially available to prevent the event [3, 17].

Educational initiatives should focus on knowledge to improve eye care of patients in ICU18 [39, 40, 47],. Training nurses based on updated clinical guidelines and eye care protocols can improve the knowledge, attitude, and practice of ICU nurses [2, 16, 17].

3. Conclusions

Corneal injury is still common in critically ill sedated and mechanically ventilated patients. The main risk factors are sedative drugs, mechanical ventilation, chemosis, lagophthalmos, and length of stay. Patients in these conditions, with altered blinking and eyelid closing reflexes, need to have their corneas lubricated with ocular gel every 6 hours and eye protection with a polyethylene chamber. Efforts should focus on education, training, and development of eye care protocols with emphasis on risk factors assessment and on the implementation of evidence-based nursing interventions.

Conflict of interest

The authors declare no conflict of interest.

Author details

Patricia R. do Prado[1*] and Fernanda R.E. Gimenes[2]

1 Federal University of Acre, Rio Branco, Acre, Brazil

2 Ribeirão Preto College of Nursing, University of São Paulo, São Paulo, Brazil

*Address all correspondence to: patyrezendeprado@gmail.com

References

[1] Barrientez B, Nicholas SE, Whelchel A, Sharif R, Hjortdal J, Karamichos D. Corneal injury: Clinical and molecular aspects. Experimental Eye Research. 2019;**186**:107709. DOI: 10.1016/j.exer.2019.107709

[2] Ebadi A, Moayed MS, Mirsadeghi A, Saeid Y. Evaluating Intensive Care nurses' clinical competence in eye Care: A cross-sectional descriptive study. Health Education and Health Promotion. 2021;**9**(3):171-175

[3] Prado PR, Silveira RCCP, Vettore MV, Fossum M, Vabo GL, Gimenes FRE. Nursing interventions to prevent corneal injury in critically ill sedated and mechanically ventilated patients: A systematic review of interventions. Intensive and Critical Care Nursing. 2023;**78**. DOI: 10.1016/j.iccn.2023.103447

[4] Standring S. Chapter 15: Development of the eye. In: Gray's Anatomy. The Anatomical Basis of Clinical Practice. 42nd Edition. Amsterdam: Elsevier; October 21, 2020. Available from: https://shop.elsevier.com/books/grays-anatomy/standring/978-0-7020-7705-0 [Accessed: July 11, 2023]

[5] Stewart S. Cornea [Internet]. 2022. Available from: https://www.kenhub.com/en/library/anatomy/cornea [Accessed: May 20, 2023]

[6] Grixti A, Sadri M, Edgar J, Datta AV. Common ocular surface disorders in patients in intensive care units. The Ocular Surface. 2012;**10**(1):26-42. DOI: 10.1016/j.jtos.2011.10.001

[7] Willmann D, Fu L, Melanson SW. Corneal Injury. Treasure Island, FL: StatPearls Publishing; 2022

[8] Silva RSCE, Gimenes FRE, Mantilla NPM, Silva NND, Pinheiro CEO, Lima MS, et al. Risk for corneal injury in intensive care unit patients: A cohort study. Intensive & Critical Care Nursing. 2021;**64**:103017. DOI: 10.1016/j.iccn.2021.103017

[9] de Oliveira Pinheiro CE, Carneiro e Silva RS, de Sousa FREG, et al. Causal validation of the risk for corneal injury in critically ill adults. Nurs Crit Care. 2022:1-8. DOI: 10.1111/nicc.12747

[10] Santos QF, Stipp MA, Góes FG, Oliveira FA, Paes GO. Incidence of corneal injury in intensive care: A cohort study. Acta Paul Enferm. 2023;36:eAPE01552. 10.37689/acta-ape/2023AO015522 [Accessed: May 20, 2023]

[11] Narmawala W, Jani HC. Exposure Keratopathy: Prophylaxys and impact of eye care education programme in ICU patients. Journal of Clinical and Diagnostic Research. 2017;11(10):6-9 10.7860/JCDR/2017/25906.10717 [Accessed: May 20, 2023]

[12] Selvan H, Pujari A, Sachan A, Gupta S, Sharma N. Neglected ocular surface care in critical care medicine: A observational study. Contact Lens & Anterior Eye. 2020;**43**(4):350-354. DOI: 10.1097/OPX.0000000000001802

[13] Alavi MN, Sharifitabar Z, Shaeri M, Hajbaghery A. An audit of eye dryness and corneal abrasion in ICU patients in Iran. Nursing in Critical Care. 2014;**19**(2):73-77. DOI: 10.1111/nicc.12052

[14] Kousha O, Kousha Z, Paddle J. Exposure keratopathy: Incidence, risk factors and impact of protocolized care on exposure keratopathy in critically

ill adults. Journal of Critical Care. 2018;**44**:413-418. DOI: 10.1016/j.jcrc.2017.11.031

[15] Freitas LS, Ferreira MA, Filho AJA, Santos CCG, Silva LB. Corneal injuries in intensive care patients: Contributions to the systematization of nursing care and patient safety. Texto & Contexto-Enfermagem. 2018;**27**(4):1-10. DOI: 10.1590/0104-07072018004960017

[16] Mehrjardi MZ, Mirzaei S, Gohari M, Hafezieh A, Nasiriani K, Luchette FA. Effect of training eye care clinical guideline for ICU patients on clinical competence of eye care in nurses. Critical Care Research Practise. 2021;**2021**:6669538. DOI: 10.1155/2021/6669538

[17] Lami S, Ayed A. Predictors of nurses' practice of eye care for patients in intensive care units. SAGE Open Nursing. 2023 Feb;**20**(9):23779608231158491. DOI: 10.1177/23779608231158491

[18] Kuruvilla S, Peter J, David S, Premkumar PS, Ramakrishna K, Thomas L, et al. Incidence and risk factor evaluation of exposure keratopathy in critically ill patients: A cohort study. Journal of Critical Care. 2015;**30**(2):400-404. DOI: 10.1016/j.jcrc.2014.10.009

[19] Sivasankar S, Jasper S, Simon S, Jacob P, John G, Raju R. Eye care in ICU. Indian Journal of Critical Care. 2006;**10**:11-14

[20] Jammal H, Khader Y, Shihadeh W, Ababneh L, AlJizawi G, AlQasem A. Exposure keratopathy in sedated and ventilated patients. Journal of Critical Care. 2012;**27**(6):537-541. DOI: 10.1016/j.jcrc.2012.02.005

[21] Werli-Alvarenga A, Ercole FF, Botoni FA, Oliveira JADMM, Chianca TCM. Corneal injuries: incidence and risk factors in the Intensive Care Unit. Rev Lat Am Enfermagem . 2011;19(5):1088-1095. Available from: https://www.scielo.br/pdf/rlae/v19n5/05.pdf [Accessed: May 20, 2023]

[22] Ho WT, Chiu CY, Chang SW. Low ambient temperature correlates with the severity of dry eye symptoms. Taiwan Journal of Ophthalmology. 2021;**12**(2):191-197. DOI: 10.4103/tjo.tjo_25_2

[23] Alven A, Lema C, Redfern RL. Impact of low humidity on damage-associated molecular patterns at the ocular surface during dry eye disease. Optometry and Vision Science. 2021;**98**(11):1231-1238. DOI: 10.1097/OPX.0000000000001802

[24] Hartford JB, Bian Y, Mathews PM, Rojas JD, Garg A, Rasool N, et al. Prevalence and risk factors for exposure keratopathy across different Intensive care units. Cornea. 2019;**38**:1124-1130. DOI: 10.1097/ICO.0000000000001961

[25] Craig JP, Nichols KK, Akpek EK, Caffery B, Dua HS, Joo CK, et al. TFOS DEWS II definition and classification report. The Ocular Surface. 2017 Jul;**15**(3):276-283. DOI: 10.1016/j.jtos.2017.05.008

[26] Fernandes APNL, Araújo JNM, Botarelli FR, Pitombeira DO, Ferreira Júnior MA, Vitor AF. Dry eye syndrome in Intensive Care units: A concept analysis. Revista Brasileira de Enfermagem. 2018;**71**(3):1162-1169. DOI: 10.1590/0034-7167-2016-0582

[27] Singh P, Gupta A, Tripathy K. Keratitis. In: StatPearls. Treasure Island (FL): StatPearls Publishing; February 22, 2023. Available from: https://www.ncbi.nlm.nih.gov/books/ NBK559014/ [Accessed: April 26, 2023]

[28] Bird B, Dingley S, Stawicki SP, Wojda TR. Exposure keratopathy in the Intensive Care unit: Do not neglect the unseen. In: Firstenberg MS, editor. Vignettes in Patient Safety. Vol. 2. London: IntechOpen; 2018. DOI: 10.5772/intechopen.72791

[29] Stepp MA, Menko AS. Immune responses to injury and their links to eye disease. Translational Research. 2021;**236**:52-71. DOI: 10.1016/j.trsl.2021.05.005

[30] Britten-Jones AC, Craig JP, Anderson AJ, Downie LE. Association between systemic omega-3 polyunsaturated fatty acid levels, and corneal nerve structure and function. Eye (Lond). 2023;**37**(9):1866-1873. DOI: 10.1038/s41433-022-02259-0

[31] Chung IY, Tavassoli S, Wong N, Cleary G. Vitamin a deficiency presenting with fungal keratitis and bilateral corneal perforations. BML Case Reports. 2022;**15**(3):e247853. DOI: 0.1136/bcr-2021-247853

[32] Ma J, Niu H, Ma X, Han C, Qu Y. Effects of long-term high-altitude exposure on retinal and choroidal microcirculation. Graefe's Archive for Clinical and Experimental Ophthalmology. 2022;**260**(11):3525-3532. DOI: 10.1007/s00417-022-05699-2

[33] Tseng CH, Tai YH, Hong CT, Dai YX, Chen TJ, Cherng YG, et al. Systemic lupus erythematosus and risk of dry eye disease and corneal surface damage: A population-based cohort study. International Journal of Environmental Research and Public Health. 2023;**20**(5):3776. DOI: 10.3390/ijerph20053776

[34] Cabrera-Aguas M, Khoo P, Watson SL. Infectious keratitis: A review. Clinical & Experimental Ophthalmology. 2022;**50**(5):543-562. DOI: 10.1111/ceo.14113

[35] Mpakosi A, Siopi M, Vrioni G, et al. Filamentous fungal keratitis in Greece: A 16-year Nationwide Multicenter survey. Mycopathologia. 2022;**187**(5-6):439-453. DOI: 10.1007/s11046-022-00666-1

[36] Lin A, Rhee MK, Akpek EK, Amescua G, Farid M, Garcia-Ferrer FJ, et al. Bacterial keratitis preferred practice pattern®. Ophthalmology. 2019;**126**(1):P1-P55. DOI: 10.1016/j.ophtha.2018.10.018

[37] Byrd LB, Martin N. Corneal Ulcer. Treasure Island (FL): StatPearls Publishing; 2022. Available from: https://www.ncbi.nlm.nih.gov/books/NBK539689/ [Accessed May 02, 2023]

[38] Kocaçal G, Eser E. Nurses can play an active role in the early diagnosis of exposure keratopathy in intensive care patients: Exposure keratopathy in intensive care units. Japan Journal of Nursing Science. 2018;**15**(1):31-38. DOI: 10.1111/jjns.12165

[39] Vyas S, Mahobia A, Bawankure S. Knowledge and practice patterns of Intensive Care unit nurses towards eye care in Chhattisgarh state. Indian Journal of Ophthalmology. 2018;**66**(9):1251-1255. DOI: 10.4103/ijo.IJO_115_18

[40] Khalil NS, Abd Elhameed SI, Abdel-kader FA, Abd Allah AA. Critical care nurses' knowledge and practices concerning eye care of patients at two teaching University Hospitals, Egypt. Nursing Healthcare International Journal. 2019;**3**(3):1-8. DOI: 10.23880/nhij-16000188

[41] Kalhori RP, Ehsani S, Daneshgar F, Ashtarian H, Rezaei M. Different nursing care methods for prevention of keratopathy among intensive care

unit patients. Global Journal of Health Science. 2015;**8**(7):212-217. DOI: 10.5539/gjhs.v8n7p212

[42] French Society for Anaesthesia and Intensive Care (SFAR); French Ophthalmology Society (SFO), French-speaking Intensive Care Society (SRLF), Keita H, et al. Eye protection in anaesthesia and intensive care. Anaesthia Critical Care Pain Medicine. 2017;**36**(6):411-418. DOI:10.1016/j.accpm.2017.08.001

[43] Ahmadinejad M, Karbasi E, Jahani Y, Ahmadipour M, Soltaninejad M, Karzari Z. Efficacy of simple eye ointment, polyethylene cover, and eyelid taping in prevention of ocular surface disorders in critically ill patients: A randomized clinical trial. Critical Care Research Practise. 2020;**2020**:6267432. DOI: 10.1155/2020/6267432

[44] Agency for Clinical Innovation (ACI). Eye Care of the Critically Ill: Clinical Practice Guide. Sydney: ACI, 2021. Available from: www.aci.health.nsw.gov.au [Accessed: April 28, 2023]

[45] Li T, Zhou H. Effect of polyethylene cover for preventing corneal injury in critically ill patients: A meta-analysis. Computational and Mathematical Methods in Medicine. 2022;**2022**:1-8. DOI: 10.1155/2022/6578229

[46] Koroloff N, Boots R, Lipman J, Thomas P, Rickard CM, Coyer F. A randomised controlled study of the efficacy of hypromellose and Lacri-Lube combination versus polyethylene/Cling wrap to prevent corneal epithelial breakdown in the semiconscious intensive care patient. Intensive Care Medicine. 2004;**30**(6):1122-1126. DOI: 10.1007/s00134-004-2203-y

[47] Güler EK, Eşer İ, Eğrilmez S. Effectiveness of polyethylene covers versus carbomer drops (Viscotears®) to prevent dry eye syndrome in the critically ill. Journal of Clinical Nursing. 2011;**20**(13-14):1916-1922. DOI: 10.1111/j.1365-2702.2010.03559.x